S0-BOK-774

Breastfeeding Annual International 2001

Breastfeeding Annual International 2001

Edited by Dia L. Michels

Foreword by Congresswoman Carolyn B. Maloney
Introduction by Lawrence M. Gartner, M.D.

PLATYPUS MEDIA LLC
WASHINGTON, DC USA
2001

For Mumsie—who carried me, suckled me, and taught me

Platypus Media is committed to the promotion and protection of breastfeeding.
We donate six percent of our profits to breastfeeding organizations.

Platypus Media LLC
627 A Street NE
Washington, DC 20002
PlatypusMedia.com
ISBN 1-930775-04-0

Edited by Where Books Begin & Irene Kleeberg Associates, New York, NY
Design by Douglas Wink, Inkway Graphics, Jersey City, NJ

Manufactured in the United States of America

Footnotes and research updates are availlable at our website, PlatypusMedia.com

Library of Congress Cataloging-in-Publication Data

The breastfeeding annual 2001 / edited by Dia L. Michels ; Foreword by
Carolyn B. Maloney ; introduction by Lawrence M. Gartner.
p. ; cm.
Includes bibliographical references and index.
ISBN: 1-930775-04-0 (alk. paper)
1. Breast feeding. 2. Infants (Newborn) — Nutrition. 3. Lactation. I.
Michaels, Dia L. II. Title
[DNLM: 1.Breast Feeding. 2. Health Promotion. WS 125 B82935 2001]
RJ216 .B7755 2001
649'.33-dc21
2001000155

Books by Dia L. Michels

MILK, MONEY, AND MADNESS
The Culture and Politics of Breastfeeding
with Naomi Baumslag, MD., M.P.H.

A WOMAN'S GUIDE TO YEAST INFECTIONS
with Naomi Baumslag, MD., M.P.H.

IF MY MOM WERE A PLATYPUS
Animal Babies And Their Mothers

ZACK IN THE MIDDLE

LOOK WHAT I SEE! WHERE CAN I BE?

Table of Contents

Section One: Getting Started

Section Two: Matters for Moms

Section Three: Breastfeeding In the Real World

Section Four: Parenting Issues

Section Five: Special Circumstances

Appendices

Acknowledgments

This book was conceived in 1997 after the success of *Milk, Money & Madness: The Culture and Politics of Breastfeeding* had created a clamor for a sequel. My determination to continue my contribution to the breastfeeding community with a second book was stymied by the many avenues open for research and discussion. Having written about the rise of the artificial formula industry, should I now concentrate on the environmental impact of breastfeeding? Or the increasingly complicated medical implications of breastfeeding in a world of prescription drugs, cancer remission, breast surgery and AIDS? Should I address the legal and practical implications of workplace breastfeeding? As I sifted through the possibilities in my mind, it dawned on me that what was needed was a single place where expertise on these myriad issues could be brought together. Thus the *Breastfeeding Annual International* was born.

While it was my inspiration that gave a structure to the book, it was the work and creativity of many hardworking people that gave it form and brought it to fruition. One constant on the journey was the energy and inspiration of La Leche League International (LLLI) leaders from all around the world. LLLI co-founder Edwina Froelich and Mary Lofton were particularly helpful. I treasure too the courage and chutzpah of LLL co-founder Marian Tompson, who is a boon companion for a long walk as well as a long talk.

There were many times I needed to clarify a topic, brainstorm an idea, or understand an issue. Again and again, I turned to James Akré at the World Health Organization's Department of Nutrition for Health and Development, and Carol Huotari, I.B.C.L.C., who manages the Center for Breastfeeding Information who were so generous with their time. Betty L. Crase, I.B.C.L.C., from the American Academy of Pediatrics was a valuable resource as were the incomparable team of Kym Smythe, I.B.C.L.C. and Terriann Shell, I.B.C.L.C.

I have been very fortunate to have assistance from a number of women who are as friendly as they are capable. Numerous tasks were taken undertaken by Carol Bruce, Gretchen Hesbacher, Henrietta Allen, B.A., M.Sc., Sandra Breisch, and Amy Condra-Peters. And, of course, there is no possibility this book would have ever been finished without the long hours and helping hands of my South African team: Karusha Moodley, Michelle Mos, Ronè Johnson and Justine Pieters.

Additionally, there are three women who probably have no idea that they generated a spark when the cinders were cooling down. Thanks for turning up the heat go to Judith M. Rovner, L.C.S.W., Meredith Small, Ph.D. and Elizabeth A. Allemann, M.D.

It has been exciting for me to bring so many voices together and hear how—as the each voice joins in—the chorus of breastfeeding advocacy grows stronger and more resonant throughout the world.

Preface

Breastfeeding is indisputably an important topic today. When I mention it to any of my Capitol Hill neighbors, whether they are lobbyists, lawyers or locals, their interest is intense. But in my work as a breastfeeding advocate, I have been continually frustrated by how scattered its constituencies are. New York Congresswoman Carolyn Maloney has introduced Federal legislation to encourage employers to support breastfeeding. Her work should impact the policies of individual states and local communities that are introducing legislation to protect women's right to breastfeed in public. Similarly, the American Academy of Pediatrics' guidelines strongly advocate that all American babies be fed only breastmilk for the first six months, and continue to breastfeed for at least the first year. One would hope that this advice would reinforce the similar recommendation recently released by the World Health Organization. With so much activity on so many levels, it is surprising that there is no single, comprehensive source for ideas and information about breastfeeding.

That is why I have compiled this anthology. I have written breastfeeding books, attended breastfeeding rallies, spoken at breastfeeding conferences and studied breastfeeding journals. I realize, however, that not everyone has the time or inclination to immerse herself to this extent, so I felt that healthcare professionals would benefit from having a single place where the latest news about breastfeeding—on every one of its fascinating fronts—could be assembled. This anthology was created to be a reliable source where experts and advocates can find out the most current information on the many facets of lactation.

For example, the legislation introducing breastfeeding into the third-grade curriculum in New York state should be of great interest to educators at all levels, from preschool through medical school. The research confirming the risks of breastmilk substitutes could be used to enrich public health programs. The importance of breastfeeding in establishing good dental health in young children should be promoted by pediatricians as well as dentists. I have tried to create a central place for information of this kind.

Breastfeeding Annual International 2001 is intended as a resource for healthcare professionals, health writers, policy makers and researchers. Its articles include medical research, legislation and policy initiatives related to breastfeeding and human lactation. Internationally known experts in the field have shared their knowledge and perspectives on issues as diverse as breastfeeding and the law, medications and breastfeeding, relactation and adoptive nursing, contraindications to breastfeeding and the costs of not breastfeeding.

As a journalist whose audience is the general public, I am less sensitive than many academics and professionals are to the criticism that social policy should not be in the same volume as medical procedures. As we learned with *Our Bodies, Ourselves* and *A Diet for a Small Planet*, the issues in nature and nurture begin with our bodies and extend outward to the ways we interact with one another and with the earth. Issues in culture and society cannot be separated from individual nutrition and child care.

Any breastfeeding mother knows that there is no point in learning how to latch on if the local laws forbid her to breastfeed her baby at the mall. There is nothing but frustration in pumping, if her school-age children learn from the formula ads that really cool moms feed baby from cans. There is no reason to go to the trouble of having a baby at a baby-friendly hospital if the doctor has prescribed mediation that is incompatible with breastfeeding.

Critics may accuse me of trying to be all things to all people. Nonetheless, I stand by my conviction that breastfeeding, like so many other issues that affect women and children, is not simply a medical matter. It is a complex issue in which policy, legislation and cultural politics play roles every bit as important as medical innovations, nursing support and education.

In compiling this anthology, I came with some preconceived notions about what would make a useful volume. I felt that it should include information on the emerging culture of attachment parenting, the new AAP guidelines and some recent developments in breastfeeding babies of HIV-positive mothers. But I was surprised by the marvelous articles that came my way, once the word was out that the anthology was coming together. The submissions gave me new insights into emerging information and what practitioners and researchers believe is important.

In keeping with the wide range and open scope of the project, I hope you will come to our website, PlatypusMedia.com, where you can contribute your thoughts about what we have done here, and suggest articles, authors and ideas for the coming volumes. Read, learn and spread the word: breast is best. If it's new and it's true, we are interested in considering it for the next volume. My goal is to produce Breastfeeding Annual International 2003, then to continue the series as an annual volume. Keeping all of us in the loop about the most current medical, political and business research and initiatives in the field will help grow and nourish the breastfeeding community to the benefit of mothers and children everywhere.

—Dia L. Michels
Washington, DC
July 2001

Through her long fight to ensure that working women throughout the United States have the right to breastfeed their children, Carolyn B. Maloney, Democratic Congresswoman from New York, has become a heroine of the breastfeeding movement. In this introduction, she explains some of the reasons behind her strong support for working women who choose to breastfeed their children

Foreword

I remember the day I told my employer I was pregnant and asked about the office's maternity policy. Their response was to call the personnel office, who told me they did not have a policy because "it had never happened before." I can still remember how terrified I was that I would lose my job

Back then, the idea of having lactation rooms at work would have seemed alien, but today we are fortunate to live in a time when breastfeeding and lactation support are becoming part of the workplace landscape. In fact, the same office I worked in now has an onsite daycare center. These changes are long overdue.

We have known for years that breastfeeding is the ideal way to feed and nurture an infant. We have known for years that it is the first line of immunization defense and that increasing breastfeeding rates leads to dramatic health benefits for both mothers and children. And we have known for years that breastfeeding does not happen by accident. New parents need support, education and encouragement to succeed at breastfeeding in a culture where bottle-feeding has been the norm for decades.

There are countries today, such as Sweden, Australia and Kenya, where almost all women begin breastfeeding after delivery, and the majority are still doing it months later. Meanwhile, the latest statistics tell us that the United States has one of the lowest breastfeeding rates of all industrialized nations and one of the highest rates of infant mortality.

Pediatricians and public health professionals around the world agree that babies should be breastfed exclusively for six months and then continue after solids are introduced for at least the first year, and longer if desired. In the U.S. today, only 61% of new mothers even attempt to breastfeed at all, and the vast majority of them have weaned before the baby is 20 weeks old. It is time for the United States to take a greater leadership role in the protection and promotion of breastfeeding.

In 2000, Dr. David Satcher, the U.S. Surgeon General, announced a new national health priority: increasing the number of U.S. women who breastfeed their babies. But many women are forced to choose between keeping their job and doing the most natural thing in the world—breastfeeding a child.

Times Have Changed

In a dramatic departure from family life in previous generations, the majority of mothers with young children are now in the workforce. Just 25 years ago, less than one-third of mothers with children under the age of one participated in the labor force. Today, almost six out of every ten women with young infants and almost 75% of mothers with children over one year of age are in the labor force. Today, it is routine for American mothers and babies to be separated during the workday.

Combine these statistics with the harsh reality that the number-one reason most women do not breastfeed or wean early is that they will be returning to the workforce after the birth of their child, and one can understand why Americans have relatively low breastfeeding rates.

Establish a Woman's Basic Rights

During the last several years, I have been working to create protections for breastfeeding on a national level, and although we face an uphill battle, we have celebrated several successes.

In 1998, Congress enacted a provision I authored allowing states to use more of their WIC (a low-income nutrition program for women, infant and children) funding for breastfeeding promotion efforts.

In 1999, Congress enacted another bill I wrote ensuring a woman's right to breastfeed while on federal property. Until then, women were being kicked out of museums, national parks and federal buildings—even the U.S. Capitol—for simply breastfeeding a child. One woman told me a park ranger told her to stop breastfeeding because "it would attract bees."

There are three more proposals still pending before Congress which would:

1. clarify the Pregnancy Discrimination Act so that it provides protection for breastfeeding women so they cannot be fired or discriminated against in the workplace for pumping breast milk or breastfeeding during their own lunch or break time;

2. create tax incentives for employers to create safe, private and clean places where women can express breast milk during the workday; and

3. establish a minimum standard to ensure that all breast pumps sold in the U.S. are safe and effective.

I also believe we should add lactation services and devices to the list of tax-deductible healthcare items under the U.S. tax code.

Breastfeeding in the Workplace

While there is general agreement that breastfeeding should be encouraged because it is good for mothers and babies, more and more companies are finding that it benefits their bottom lines. Support for breastfeeding in the workplace has been shown to lower healthcare costs, enhance productivity, improve employee satisfaction, increase retention of workers and improve a corporate image. No doubt, raising breastfeeding rates in America is a win-win proposition.

Many companies have discovered these benefits for themselves. And interestingly, many of them are insurance companies that know which policies help keep down healthcare costs.

In the first year of its corporate lactation program, Aetna, Inc., estimated it saved $1,435 in medical claims and three days of sick leave per breastfed baby. That was a total savings to them of $108,737 in 1997—an almost three-to-one return on investment in claims alone. Other companies such as Bankers Trust, Cigna, Kellogg's, Chase Manhattan Bank, Eastman Kodak, PricewaterhouseCoopers and Electronic Data Systems have all found that promoting breastfeeding is good for business.

Getting Involved

When women first started calling my office complaining that they were being fired because they used their own lunch times or break times to express breast milk, I simply could not believe it. But sadly, the more research I did, the more I found that breastfeeding was being discouraged in many ways in our country.

Employees can take lunch breaks, coffee breaks—even smoking breaks—and no one says a word. But those who used that time to provide optimal nutrition for a child were facing problems.

As an active member and former Co-Chair of the Congressional Caucus for Women's Issues, I felt obliged to help these women who faced discrimination and harassment for doing the most natural thing in the world—feeding a child.

One lactating woman said a man had presented his coffee cup to her and asked for some milk. Another had a coworker outside her office moo-ing while she pumped milk during her lunch break. And yet another was told "we don't want that kind of thing on our premises."

More and more women told me that they were fired, while the courts unevenly ruled that lactation was not "a condition related to pregnancy" and therefore not covered by current anti-discrimination laws. My friends, if breastfeeding is not related to pregnancy, I don't know what is!

Some women complained that they bought breast pumps that were painful and ineffective. Many women told me they gave up breastfeeding after using sub-standard breast pumps, blaming themselves for failing to express milk. Little did they know that although we have minimum standards in place for everything from stethoscope to blood pressure machines to thermometers, when it comes to breast pumps you take your chances with what you buy. No minimum standards exist for breast pumps; anybody can sell you anything.

It has been heartening to learn that businesses—large and small—are getting into the act, putting lactation programs in place for their new moms. Many employers around the country have called me to say they want to help; they want to support their new moms who choose to breastfeed. However, not every woman is fortunate enough to work for such an employer.

As long as women are facing discrimination and being harassed for choosing to breastfeed a child, I will continue to work on their behalf.

The Need for Federal Legislation

Several states have enacted laws to protect the nursing mother from charges of indecency or grant her the right to nurse where and when she wishes. But the economic, social and health benefits of encouraging breastfeeding are far too important to be left to a patchwork of legislation that varies from county to county, state to state.

Federal laws are needed to give today's families and tomorrow's leaders the opportunity to have the best possible start in life. Our children—and certainly the future of the health of our nation—depend on it.

—Carolyn B. Maloney
Washington, DC
July 2001

Congresswoman Carolyn B. Maloney, a Democrat, represents the 14th district in New York City, an area that contains many of the city's most historic and well-known neighborhoods. After serving on the New York City Council for ten years (and becoming the first council member to give birth while in office) she was elected to Congress in 1992 and reelected in 2000 with 73% of the vote. She served as Co-Chair of the Women's Caucus during the 106th Congress and continues to be a leading advocate for women, children and family issues. Her website has a wealth of information on the benefits of breastfeeding, the cost-savings to the nation and the status of her legislative efforts.

In 1997 the American Academy of Pediatrics issued a policy statement recommending breastfeeding for all babies, including premature and sick babies (see Appendices). Lawrence M. Gartner, M.D., was chairman on the Work Group on Breastfeeding of the A.A.P., which led the publication of this statement. In this foreword Dr. Gartner explains why breastfeeding is always worth the effort.

Introduction
What Only a Woman Can Do—Breastfeed

Anyone can change a baby's diaper, rock a baby to sleep and take a baby for a walk, but just as only a woman can produce a child, so too, only a woman can provide that child with the perfect food: breast milk. Breastfeeding is a perfectly natural act, but like other natural events, such as menopause, it may prove more difficult for some women than others. Nevertheless, it is always worth the effort because of its overwhelming benefits to both mother and baby.

People working with new mothers at all levels of health care should be aware of the importance of breastfeeding to ensure that mothers do not see it as one of two choices but as the best choice and, when possible, the only choice.

The Medical View

After a period during which only lip service was often given to the saying "breast is best," the people who know about the subject of breastfeeding from a medical perspective—pediatricians, obstetricians and family doctors—agree that breast milk is best for babies, including premature and sick babies. In the past, doctors only recommended breast milk for full-term babies with no health problems.

Now, since December 1997, the American Academy of Pediatrics in a policy statement written by the Work Group on Breastfeeding, of which I was chairman, recommends breast milk for infants born prematurely, and also those with a variety of illnesses including respiratory and infectious diseases as well as potential hindrances to breastfeeding such as cleft palate and Down syndrome.

These guidelines, which the American Academy of Pediatrics points out reflect "the considerable advances that have occurred in recent years in the scientific knowledge of the benefits of breastfeeding, in the mechanisms underlying these benefits and in the practice of breastfeeding," urge "Enthusiastic support and involvement of pediatricians in the promotions and practice of breastfeeding" and that babies, including premature ones, should be exclusively breastfed for 6 months, then breastfed in combination with solid food for at least another 6 months—one full year or longer.

As pediatricians, we recommend this because breast milk not only provides an infant with the calories and fluid it needs for growth and development, but also provides significant protection against chronic diseases such as asthma and lymphoma, and infectious diseases including diarrhea, ear infections, meningitis, and pneumonia. The immune components of breast milk constantly change to meet the infant's needs to be protected against new infections.

Breast milk is what the newborn needs—and in nearly all cases it is all that the newborn needs for about the first six months of life. Therefore, it is vitally important for mothers to begin breastfeeding in the hospital or pumping to provide breast milk even if the infant cannot breastfeed directly.

Off to a Good Start

Those doctors and other caregivers who have worked for years with breastfeeding mothers and their new babies know the major importance of getting breastfeeding off to a good start. The AAP recommends that breastfeeding begin within the first hour of birth. The AAP guidelines emphasize that no water, glucose water or infant formula should be given to a breastfeeding newborn unless there are specific medical indications. Mothers should provide expressed breast milk for times when they are separated from their new babies because of infant or maternal illness. In order to assist mothers who must express milk, hospitals should provide quality breast pumps to such mothers.

Once a mother goes home, she is in a world that uses the baby bottle as the universal symbol of infant feeding. Mothers, most of whom are not trained in the physiology, biochemistry and immunology of breast milk, may believe from exposure to advertising that using infant formula is safer, more sterile and more convenient than breastfeeding.

The Superiority of Human Milk

This is far from the truth, and it is a major responsibility of those working with new mothers to help them understand that the breastfeeding mother is giving her child a product any knowledgeable doctor can guarantee is superior to the best infant formula. Human milk, offering as it does complete nutrition for babies—including hormones and antibodies compared to factory produced formula—is also efficient in its packaging! It is clean, fresh and warm and can't be forgotten and left somewhere. There are no labels to check, no bottles to sterilize, no measuring, no timing.

And the benefits of breast milk last well beyond infancy. Children, adolescent, and adults who were breastfed as infants generally tend to have better health profiles than those who were not.

Benefits to the Mother

There is a tendency for those who write about breastfeeding to emphasize its benefits to the baby, but there are also many benefits to the mother. Mothers who breastfeed recover more quickly from childbirth with reduced postpartum blood loss and an earlier return to pre-pregnancy weight. Mothers who breastfeed often also enjoy a lengthy absence of menstruation.

While this time without ovulation—known as lactation amenorrhea—cannot be used reliably for birth control beyond the early months of exclusive breastfeeding, it does offer advantages for women's health. It reduces the iron loss a woman experiences in menstruation, lowering her risk for iron-deficiency anemia.

We also know that women who have breastfed have lower risks of ovarian and breast cancers, as well as osteoporosis. There is speculation that prolonging the period of estrogen suppression, as occurs during pregnancy and lactation, protects against these hormonally dependent diseases. Breastfeeding is also to play a part in building the bonding relationship between mother and child, although the same bonding can occur with a bottle-fed baby.

Reduced Healthcare Costs

Because of these advantages to both mother and baby, breastfeeding results in reduced healthcare costs. Many businesses support breastfeeding because they have found that it reduces worker absenteeism—mothers don't have to stay home as often because their breastfed babies are less susceptible to childhood illnesses.

There are practical barriers to breastfeeding, and those advising mothers should be aware of them and be sympathetic about them. A mother may not start to breastfeed because she plans on returning to work as soon as possible. A mother whose partner is away a lot may be afraid her child will be too dependent on her if she breastfeeds.

The mother returning to work can continue to breastfeed as more states and even the federal government are writing laws to protect pumping and even breastfeeding in workplaces. Some companies have lactation consultants on their staffs and special rooms and equipment for mothers who pump. And psychological studies have shown that breastfeeding enhances the child's sense of being loved and nurtured. Breastfeeding, especially when continued into the second and even third year of life, may increase the child's independence and self-assurance.

Best for Baby, Best for Mother

Far too often, breastfeeding is presented to pregnant women and new mothers as little more than one feeding option, only marginally different from formula-feeding. This is wrong. Breast milk is radically different from infant formula, both nutritionally and for its growth and anti-infectious properties.

Nutritionally, the protein and fat in breast milk are entirely different from formula. Certain fats in human milk that have been shown to be critical in brain development are absent from formulas. Although the main carbohydrate, lactose, is the same in both human milk and formula, human milk contains hundreds of specialized complex carbohydrates that protect the bowel from diseases and toxins. Growth factors in human milk promote intestinal and other organs to mature more rapidly.

Immunologically breast milk supplies antibodies and other anti-infectious agents that are entirely absent in commercial formula. The bacteria in the intestine of a breastfed baby are different and less pathogenic than those of an artificially fed infant, suppressing growth of *E. coli* and other pathogens.

Emotionally, breastfeeding and bottle-feeding are very different experiences for both the baby and the mother. And it's not just pediatricians who are enthusiastically supporting breastfeeding. Other professionals involved in infant health are strongly committed to breastfeeding. The American College of Obstetricians and Gynecologists (ACOG), in conjunction with the American Academy of Pediatrics (AAP), is jointly working to develop policies and educational materials to support and assure optimal healthcare outcomes for pregnant women and their children.

Recently, the Academy of Breastfeeding Medicine (ABM), the only multi-specialty medical society dedicated to breastfeeding, has provided a forum for obstetricians, gynecologists, pediatricians, family practitioners, surgeons and preventive medicine physicians to discuss and develop breastfeeding education and promotion initiatives, as well as clinical research. In the United States, medical schools have recently added courses on breastfeeding and infant nutrition. For those of us who have been in the forefront of this movement, it is deeply satisfying to look back and see what strides medicine and activist mothers have made together to provide the best for babies.

The Parents' Choice

Parents have the right to choose any nourishment they like for their baby. Advice will come from formula manufacturers, in-laws, helpful neighbors and friends. But obstetricians and pediatricians who have kept up-to-date on their training will always say that breastfeeding is the healthiest alternative.

As scientists as well as clinicians, they know that there really isn't any equivalent to human milk. Baby formulas are clearly inferior. In fact, the World Health Organization rates infant formula as the fourth most desirable infant food, after breast milk from the mother, breast milk from another woman and donor milk from a human milk bank. Is it any surprise that most educated women choose to breastfeed?

In the United States, 74 % of college-educated women breastfeed their newborns, while only 43 % of mothers with a grade-school education do the same. Breastfeeding education is a wise investment of a mother's time. Women who choose to breastfeed need to discuss this with their physicians to be sure there will be knowledgeable and committed support for this decision. A mother should tell her obstetrician that she is committed to initiating breastfeeding and ask that her baby be put to her breast immediately after birth and certainly within the first hour.

She should check that her hospital will provide her with rooming-in around the clock, enforce a no-bottle policy and provide access to a staff lactation consultant.

She should ask her pediatrician to help her overcome the obstacles she may encounter in breastfeeding and be certain the pediatrician is knowledgeable regarding breastfeeding management and will be truly supportive.

She may want to contact a local La Leche League International chapter and get a list of nearby lactation consultants (look for ones that have "IBCLC" after their name). Joining an LLLI group will also provide peer support, not just on breastfeeding but also on other aspects of child care.

Finally, she will want to review her insurance plan to see if it covers breastfeeding support. For women who participate in WIC, the local office should be able to provide resources to ensure lactation success. Advice from well-trained caregivers is a good antidote for the old wives' tales that mothers encounter as they raise their children.

You have just begun this book. Read on, and you will understand why so many of us have become committed to working together to see that as many children as possible begin and continue their lives on the best infant food, human milk.

—Lawrence M. Gartner, MD
Valley Center, CA
July 2001

Lawrence M. Gartner, M.D., Professor Emeritus, Department of Pediatrics and Obstetics/Gynecology, University of Chicago, chaired the committee that led to the adoption by the American Academy of Pediatrics of its Policy Statement on Breastfeeding and the Use of Human Milk which set standard practice for the field. In addition to serving on many other important committees, he was a member of the group which produced, also for the AAP, practice guidelines for the Management of Hyperbilirubinemia in the Healthy Term Newborn. He is also past President of the Academy of Breastfeeding Medicine and Founding Editor of its newsletter *ABM News & Views*. Dr. Gartner has recently taken on the responsibility of organizing the new AAP Section on Breastfeeding.

Section One

Getting Started

Jack Newman, M.D., estimates that he has helped 15,000 women breastfeed their children. It is important that the breastfeeding mother not feel she is alone in a commercial, bottle-feeding world. This chapter discusses ways in which the breastfeeding mother can be helped to withstand pressures that may encourage her to "give up."

Chapter 1

Helping the Breastfeeding Mother

Jack Newman, M.D., F.R.C.P.C.

When a mother decides to breastfeed her baby, she is carrying on a tradition that has continued *almost* uninterrupted since the beginning of mammalian life on earth, some 200 million years ago, give or take a few million. Not only that, of course, she is also doing the best for her baby and for herself, because no artificial baby milk (formula) has even come close to breast milk in duplicating the variety of ingredients and the complexity of the interaction of these ingredients.

There are hundreds of ingredients present in breast milk that have specific functions and are not present in artificial baby milk, despite what the formula makers try to make you believe. And breastfeeding is not simply breast milk. It is an entire behavior, a special relationship between the mother and her child that is more than breast milk—in the same way that love is more than sex.

Almost uninterrupted? Almost. Until about 150 years ago, almost all babies were breastfed, although not necessarily by their own mothers. In some societies, especially in Europe, the mothers of aristocratic and even middle-class families often did not breastfeed, giving their babies away to wet nurses to feed. It was, of course, a sign of status to be able to pay others to do things for you—gardening, cooking, feeding your child, even raising your child. Showing that you are above the common herd seems to be important for many people. Furthermore, the birth spacing effects of breastfeeding—largely forgotten in our day and age—were well known in those times, and aristocratic families wanted to have many children, so that breastfeeding by the mother was definitely discouraged among members of the nobility. Generally, until the past century and a half, almost all babies in the world were breastfed, sometimes for several years in many societies. Only in a few societies was milk other than human milk used to feed small babies.

BUSINESS STEPS IN

Then, business started getting interested in selling milk to mothers. There was a market—a lucrative one as it turned out. With the Industrial Revolution, people moved to the cities and more and more women went to work in factories, their work there preventing breastfeeding their babies the way they did when they worked in and around their homes in rural areas. Women lost touch with the traditions of breastfeeding and depended more and more on "professionals" to guide them with childcare, including infant feeding. So more and more women began using breast-milk substitutes. Marketing techniques have changed, but the message of the manufacturers has always been the same: "Our milk is almost the same as mother's milk." This is the message now, and it was the message 100 years ago, when we hardly knew what was in breast milk. The message is just as wrong today as it was 100 or more years ago.

At about the same time as business became interested in infant feeding, so did the medical profession—for both altruistic and financial reasons. There was always the problem of how to feed orphaned babies. In some societies orphaned babies were nursed by relatives of the mother. Orphanages often hired wet nurses, but often there were not enough available to feed all the orphans. Also, what were the factory workers going to feed their babies, if indeed they were able to feed them while they worked? There seemed to be no question of maternity leave in this money-driven society, or, except rarely, having day care on the premises of the mothers' work.

Feeding straight animal milk, of course, was often associated with severe illness and death of the baby, either because the milk was not clean for lack of refrigeration, or infected with tuberculosis, or the ingredients were unsuitable for human infants or were present in too large or too small quantities. As well, milk was often fatal because it was diluted with water, or the cream was skimmed off by the unscrupulous, who were trying to make a little more money.

So physicians began to become involved and tried to make infant feeding "scientific," by studying the ingredients of human milk and trying to adapt animal milk to the needs of infants. Cow's milk became the main source for the base of the milk that was "adapted" for babies, not because it had any special properties, but simply because it was the most abundant and least expensive. Physicians became wealthy by inventing their own formulas, but most of them saw a new source of income from patients coming to see them to help them with infant feeding. In those days, women would never have imagined going to a physician (almost all of whom were men) for advice about breastfeeding. But with the advent of artificial feeding, they became dependent upon physicians for guidance.

By the 1920s, artificial feeding was no longer a rarity, and a cozy relationship had developed between the medical profession and the manufacturers of artificial milks for babies that has continued to this day. The formula companies agreed to encourage mothers to go to physicians to get advice about infant feeding, and not advertise directly to the public (though this part of the understanding has fallen by the wayside recently), while physicians helped market the new products. By the 1950s many physicians truly believed that artificial feeding was better than breastfeeding, because it was "more scientific." By the early 1970s, artificial feeding had become the rule, the model by which both lay people and health professionals understood infant feeding. Unfortunately, even in the 1990s, despite an upsurge in breastfeeding in the affluent world starting some fifteen years earlier, the formula-fed baby and formula-feeding mother were still considered the model for infant feeding, and breastfeeding babies and mothers were generally forced to conform to this model—often with disastrous consequences for the breastfeeding relationship.

So what should every breastfeeding mother know? She needs to know that what's true about bottle-feeding is not necessarily true about breastfeeding. She needs to know that many of the people who will be advising her—relatives, friends and health professionals—understand breastfeeding only in terms of artificial feeding and that they understand artificial feeding much better than they do breastfeeding. She needs to know that very few health professional—*especially* pediatricians—acquire even the rudiments of breastfeeding during their training, and even fewer have had any practical training. She needs to know, also, that because many health professionals or their wives did not breastfeed their own babies, too many of them feel justified in not being supportive of breastfeeding—though they may *say* they are.

Luckily, things are changing, although slowly, and the health professionals a mother encounters may be extremely supportive and helpful. But the breastfeeding mother should be wary. She needs to know that if everything goes well with her breastfeeding, as it often does, everyone will support it. But if her breastfeeding is not going so well, she may be bombarded with advice to stop or supplement—despite the fact that usually a little knowledgeable advice will help overcome even seemingly insoluble problems. And finally, she needs to know that she may be deluged by free samples of formula and "educational" materials from formula companies and their health-professional collaborators who say they support

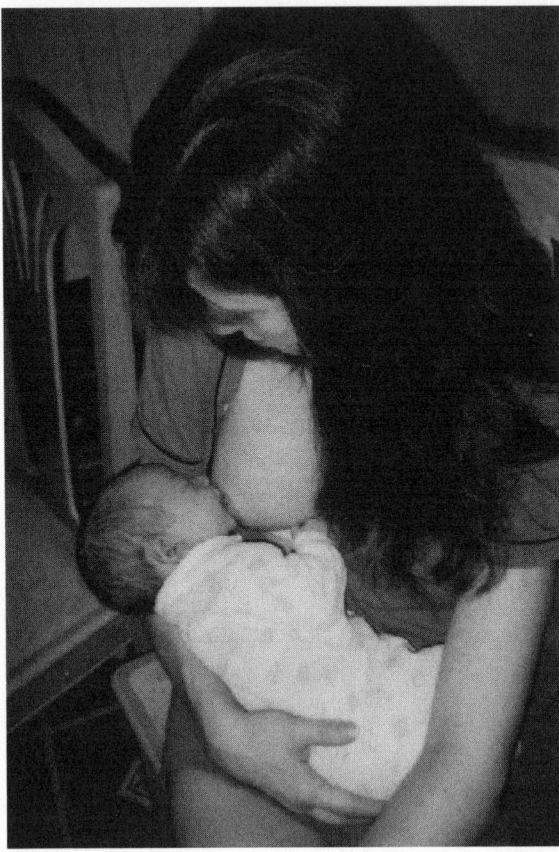

Supervision of the latching-on process is crucial to the successful initiation of breastfeeding. When the baby's chin first touches the mother's breast, she can point her nipple toward the back of his mouth, so that he can get as much milk as he needs. His mouth should close around both the nipple and the aureole.

breastfeeding. She should never forget there is only one purpose for sending her samples and "educational" materials: so that she will buy the products.

What are some examples of how the *artificially fed baby* is used as the model for infant feeding and forcing this model on the *breastfeeding baby*?

"There Is No Milk in the First Few Days"

On the very first day, the mother may be told that her baby needs to be supplemented. Though this is very rarely necessary, most of the time this has more to do with the fact that formula-fed babies will take a lot more from a bottle than breastfed babies get from their mother's breasts in the first couple of days. Instead of making the correct deduction—that formula-fed babies are drinking *too* much—it is often assumed there is not enough milk in the first few days; it is as if the formula-fed baby sets the standard.

But if there is enough, why do so many breastfed babies seem to want to feed so much in the first few days? Because the baby who is not latched on well has difficulty getting milk, *especially* when the supply is not abundant. Once the supply is abundant, the baby may get milk very well, even with a poor latch-on, though there is often a price to pay—sore nipples, long, frequent feedings, blocked ducts, colicky baby. Unfortunately, many (but not all) of our postpartum staff are so lacking in breastfeeding training that the mother may be told the baby's latch-on is very good when it is not. One of the best ways of judging whether or not the latch is good is by the degree of the mother's pain in breastfeeding. In the first few days, many mothers do experience some nipple tenderness, but severe pain is not normal and is almost always due to latch-on.

"There Is No Such Thing as Nipple Confusion"

You can almost always force a baby to take a bottle nipple, though to do so eventually becomes difficult if the baby breastfeeds well. But even strong breastfeeding advocates will argue this point. The fact of the matter is that babies are not stupid. They want milk, and they will go to where the milk is found. And if they do not get it easily from the breast, but get it well from a bottle, they will prefer the bottle. Why might they not get it easily from the breast? Because breastfeeding is hard work for the baby? No, it isn't. But if the baby is not latched on well, he may not get milk easily. When a baby latches on poorly, it is—to use an analogy easily understood in our bottle-feeding society—similar to giving him a bottle with a nipple hole that is too small; the bottle is full, but the baby will not easily get the milk from it. However, when a mother has an abundant supply and the baby drinks well at the breast, he may accept both breast and bottle well.

There are now, however, valuable methods of supplement, if supplementation is truly necessary, which do not require a bottle. If there are alternatives, why not use them instead? Because the bottle is *natural*? It says volumes about our society that so many people find the bottle natural, and a cup or nursing supplementer unnatural.

"Babies Need to Feed X Number of Times a Day for Y Minutes"

This belief is a perfect example of how even breastfeeding advocates can get confused. The concern is not how often or how long a baby is at the breast, but rather how well he feeds. A baby who feeds well five times a day is better off than a baby who feeds poorly ten times a day. A baby may be "at the breast" but not actually getting milk. A baby who drinks at the breast for twenty minutes is getting a lot more milk than a baby who drinks for two minutes but then sucks without getting milk for two more hours. The better the latch-on, the more likely a baby is to get milk during a longer part of the feeding.

"Jaundice Is Bad and Requires the Interruption of Breastfeeding"

Actually it is almost never necessary or desirable to interrupt breastfeeding because of jaundice. Jaundice, which is due to the rapid, abnormal destruction of the baby's blood cells, often resulted, in the past, in serious injury or even death for the baby, but this is different from what most babies are now experiencing. Although cases of abnormal jaundice still occur, the majority of cases of jaundice in the breastfed baby are due, at least in the first three or four days after birth, to an *inadequate intake* of breast milk. The approach to dealing with this is to fix the breastfeeding so that it results in adequate feeding, not stop the breastfeeding.

If you look carefully at any exclusively breastfed baby, you will see that even at six or eight weeks of life, chances are he is still slightly yellow (jaundiced). Because this is common, and breastfeeding is, after all, the normal, physiologic method of feeding, jaundice is normal. What's not normal is the absence of jaundice in artificially fed babies. We don't believe that this absence of jaundice harms the artificially fed baby. The so-called "prolonged" jaundice of the breastfed infant is not a reason to interrupt breastfeeding even for a single feeding. If, however, there is an abnormality causing the jaundice, it is extremely unusual that stopping breastfeeding, even temporarily, would be required or helpful. In such a situation, the abnormality is treated, and the breastfeeding is not interrupted.

"When a Baby or His Mother Is Sick, It Is Better Not to Breastfeed"

On the contrary, when the baby or his mother is sick, breastfeeding is more important than ever. It may not always be possible, because of the severity of the illness, but that does not diminish the importance of breastfeeding. Health professionals or hospitals that have enlightened policies will do all they can to encourage the continuation of breastfeeding, and it is amazing what can be arranged even in very difficult circumstances. Premature babies need breast milk, and breastfeeding, more, not less. Babies who have diarrhea need breastfeeding more, not less. Mothers who have mastitis should breastfeed their babies on the affected side so that the mastitis resolves more quickly. Mothers who take medication can almost always continue breastfeeding, because most drugs come out into the milk in such tiny quantities that they are extremely unlikely to be clinically significant for the baby. Drugs of concern usually have an alternative that can be used safely. A physician who is supportive of breastfeeding will make every effort to prescribe medication that is compatible with it.

Myths and misinformation abound, sometimes propagated by people very supportive of, but not knowledgeable about, breastfeeding. A mother may or may not be so fortunate as to have a supportive milieu and supportive health professionals. Remember, then, that breastfeeding is not simply "preferred," it is best for the mother and for the baby. The substitutes for breastfeeding are no better than adequate—and for too many babies, inadequate. Supplementation is occasionally necessary, but not as often as suggested. Many health professionals do not know how to help, even when they would like to. But more and more help is available, and more and more physicians, nurses, and lactation consultants are developing the expertise to help even when problems seem insurmountable.

Jack Newman, M.D., has worked throughout the world as a pediatrician. His home in Toronto, Canada, is his base, but he has practiced medicine in places as diverse as Latin America and South Africa. "When you work in places that have very few resources," explains Dr. Newman, "you learn to distill medicine down to its most basic elements." In 1984, Newman established the first breastfeeding clinic in Toronto. Today he runs four clinics in Canada. But he hasn't given up his love of travel. He continues to travel the globe, teaching medical professionals how to support and counsel breastfeeding women. His latest book is *Dr. Jack Newman's Guide to Breastfeeding* (HarperCollins, Canada), also titled *The Ultimate Book of Breastfeeding Answers* (Prima, U.S.).

In most parts of the world, breastfeeding is treated as being absolutely normal—which it is. But in our commercialized, industrialized culture, it may seem more complicated. This chapter discusses some of the issues that may face today's breastfeeding mother, and suggests ways to help her prepare to solve problems.

Chapter 2
Preparing for Nursing

Gale Pryor

One of the best ways in which a health professional can help a new mother is by being ready to assist her with any questions or problems she may have with breastfeeding her baby. That is why we are placing this chapter here, so that after discussing the basics we can return to the fundamental truth that breastfeeding is about a woman—one woman—and her relationship to her baby.

Ask a pregnant woman who lives on the plains of Africa or on an atoll in the South Pacific how she is preparing to breastfeed her baby, and she will be puzzled by the question. After all, what is she supposed to be doing that her body is not already doing on its own? When the baby is born, she will put him to her breast. Soon her milk will be ready, and the baby will nurse and grow—and that will be that. What could possibly be simpler? In North America and other, more developed parts of the world, breastfeeding can be that simple but often is not. Both breastfeeding and giving birth in our industrialized, medicalized culture have been complicated by "improvements" that too often, in the end, interfere with a process already honed to perfection by thousands and thousands of years of human physical and behavioral evolution.

In addition, the rarity with which we see mothers nursing babies prevents mothers from learning about breastfeeding as they do in other cultures, by observation. Children in these cultures grow up being breastfed and with breastfed babies all around them. When the girls grow up and have their own babies, they are well prepared to nurse them. Like chimpanzees raised in captivity—who have never seen another chimp with a nursing baby, and who must be shown by their human caretakers how to hold and feed theirs—most American mothers have missed out on a basic part of their mothering education. In primates, including humans, breastfeeding is learned rather than instinctual.

LEARNING ABOUT BREASTFEEDING

Familiarizing herself with breastfeeding, therefore, is the most essential way in which a mother can prepare herself to nourish and nurture her baby. She should learn as much as she can about how her breasts make milk, why human milk is the perfect food for the human baby, how babies nurse, and what she needs to know in the first days of nursing her baby. She should read up-to-date, trusted books about breastfeeding, but also be sure to find other women who have successfully and happily nursed their babies. Spending time with nursing mothers and babies will enable her to observe and learn—as she was meant to do—how mothers hold their babies, how the babies settle into a nursing or signal that they've finished, and how long and how often a baby might breastfeed.

If no one in her circle of friends or family is nursing a baby, the mother should try to attend a local La Leche League group's monthly meetings, where she will be surrounded by nursing couples and her questions will be welcomed. An international organization of nursing mothers dedicated to helping other nursing mothers, La Leche League can be an invaluable resource for accurate and empathetic breastfeeding advice and support. The mother may also wish to attend a breastfeeding class, if her hospital or doctor's office offers one. Ideally, experienced mothers not only can demonstrate much of what the mother will need to know, but will also become a valuable source of information and support after the baby is born.

FINDING SUPPORT

Just as humans were intended to learn about breastfeeding from others, so are we meant to care for our newborns with the assistance of others. As one anthropologist has said, "It is biologically inappropriate for humans to care for babies in isolation." Before the baby is born, mothers should seek out people who will be supportive of breastfeeding and will be most helpful when her newborn is brought home. Mothers should encourage the baby's father, often the steadiest support, to learn as much about breastfeeding as possible as well, so that he will trust and take pride in the mother's body's ability to nourish the baby.

If the baby's father does not live with the mother, or is doubtful about breastfeeding, other sources of support will become imperative. A *doula*, or mother's helper, can be invaluable. Agencies are cropping up to provide *doula*s who can give general help and informed breastfeeding support for the first week or two

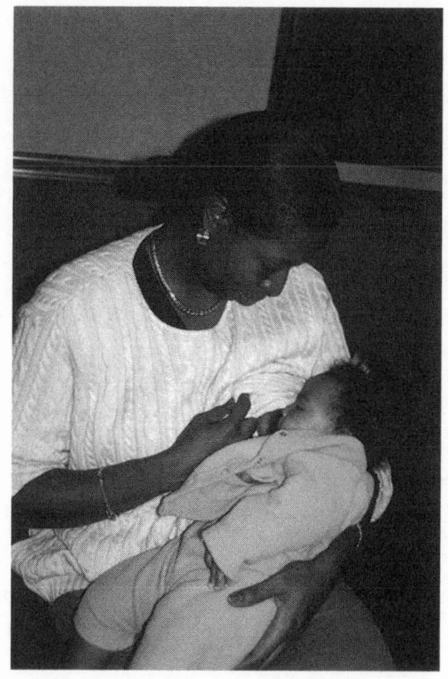

To initiate the very first breastfeeding, the mother—the baby cuddled in her arms—may need forty-eight hours to lactate. The baby's presence is by no means insignificant to the lactating, but contributes to it.

after a baby comes home. The added cost of hiring a *doula* pays for itself in the guarantee of a good start to nursing and mothering. The name and number of a certified lactation consultant—a professional who specializes in diagnosing and resolving nursing problems—can be a godsend. Mothers may wish to visit with a nearby lactation consultant even before the baby is born to discuss any concerns they may have. Lactation consultants often rent out breast pumps, as well as give advice, and can be invaluable sources of information for mothers planning to return to work.

Mothers should decide early whom they will call for encouragement and help: a neighbor, a friend, a professional *doula*, a lactation consultant, a La Leche League leader, a relative, or anyone who is knowledgeable and enthusiastic about breastfeeding. It is likely that all will go smoothly, but knowing that help is there if needed will free the mother to relax and enjoy her new nursing baby without fretting.

CHOOSING A HOSPITAL

Most breastfeeding complications can be prevented altogether if a mother is given the right information and assisted in truly helpful ways in the first hours and days of her baby's life. The care the mother and her baby receive in the hospital may spell the difference between a smooth start and a rocky one. If a mother's health insurance allows her to choose the hospital where she will give birth, and she lives in an area where a number of choices are available, she may be able to find a hospital known for its progressive maternity policies. If her choices are more limited, she may need to work with her obstetrician and the hospital administration in advance to ensure her preferences are met.

The best start to breastfeeding is one that keeps mother and baby close to each other from birth on, day and night, to allow unlimited breastfeedings. An ideal beginning would be free of inaccurate advice and critical comments. A few key questions to the obstetrician and the maternity ward nursing staff will help a mother find out if this is a hospital where it is possible to begin breastfeeding comfortably.

QUESTIONS TO ASK

The mother should ask if she will be able to nurse her baby immediately after the baby's birth—even if she has a cesarean delivery. The first minutes after birth offer an optimal opportunity (although not the only one) for a mother and baby to establish breastfeeding—and a strong attachment. Babies display a readiness to suckle during the first two hours after birth that is not as strong again until forty hours later.

If a mother nurses soon after birth, her baby's breastfeeding will help contract her uterus by stimulating release of the hormone oxytocin. A good beginning to breastfeeding for the baby, this first nursing also heralds the mother's recovery from birth. Although most hospitals no longer routinely separate mothers and babies after birth, mothers may still need to state firmly their preferences on the matter. Mothers must let the doctor and the hospital staff know that they intend to nurse as soon as possible after giving birth, whether in the delivery room after a vaginal birth or in the recovery room after a cesarean section.

The mother should ask whether the hospital allows "rooming in," or keeping the baby with her in her room on the maternity ward rather than in the central nursery. She should find out if she needs to arrange a private room in advance in order to be allowed to keep her baby with her at all times. Full-time rooming-in allows a mother to feed her baby whenever and for however long both wish, day and night, which is the very best way to guarantee a bountiful milk supply and avoid engorgement. If the hospital routinely gives babies bottles of sugar water in the nursery—a practice that interferes with successful breastfeeding—keeping the baby in the mother's room will prevent this. Keeping the baby with the mother also means that she will know him better and feel more confident caring for him when the time comes to leave the hospital.

NIGHT NURSING

Nursing at night is especially important for establishing breastfeeding. Prolactin, one of the milk-making hormones, increases during the nighttime. Nursing off and on during these hours keeps the milk supply high, even if nursing decreases during the day. In fact, in cultures where breastfeeding is the norm it is unheard of for a very young baby to sleep anywhere other than in his mother's arms. Not only is it the most comfortable, secure place for a baby, but it is also the easiest way to breastfeed as frequently as a newborn requires.

Simply putting the baby, already cuddled in the mother's arms, to her breast and then falling back to sleep as he nurses is far more restful than being wakened by a nurse with a hungry baby in her arms, sitting up, nursing, and ringing the nurse to come back for the baby (who may well be wide awake after all this activity). In general, sleep and nursing patterns that are comfortable for both mother and baby develop fastest when mother and baby stay together, day and night, from birth on.

If a mother is bound to a hospital that has a firm policy of keeping babies in the nursery while their mothers are asleep, the mother may find that, once she is on the maternity ward, she can circumvent it by politely refusing the nurses' offers to take her baby to the nursery. If on occasion they prevail and the baby does spend some part of the night in the nursery, the mother should state firmly that the baby is to be brought to her as soon as he is awake—well before he begins to fuss.

Mothers should inquire whether the hospital has a lactation consultant on staff, for the breastfeeding advice given by the staff may be more accurate, on the whole, than on wards without a lactation consultant. Before or after they give birth, mothers should also ask about the availability of breastfeeding classes or videotapes before or after they give birth. In any case, the mother should plan to bring her most trusted breastfeeding reference to the hospital with her so that she can rely on it for answers to questions. While many maternity nurses are well informed and current on breastfeeding, a few continue to dispense blatantly poor advice. The time limits per side for each breastfeeding advocated by many nurses, for example, are a sure recipe for reduced milk supply, poor weight gain, and sore nipples. Without dismissing everything a mother learns in the hospital, she still may wish to double-check any recommendations about breastfeeding in a respected book at her bedside.

CHOOSING A PEDIATRICIAN

Regardless of whether the mother's hospital experience is optimal or not, it will always be short. Her relationship with her pediatrician, however, may last for years and years. While the American Academy of Pediatricians has gone on record as supporting the breastfeeding of babies for from one to two years, the fact is that many pediatricians are still not thoroughly trained in lactation and breastfeeding support. While any pediatrician a mother speaks to will probably support her decision to breastfeed, not every pediatrician is going to be as helpful as she might hope. A mother should consider interviewing a family practice physician, who will care for both the mother and her baby. A nursing couple is a dyad; it makes sense for them to be treated by the same doctor. In addition, family physicians are rapidly gaining a reputation for being better informed and helpful about breastfeeding than specialists in pediatrics or obstetrics.

A few carefully phrased questions may assist in flushing out those doctors who are not only enthusiastic but also truly knowledgeable and experienced. The mother should ask first how many of that doctor's patients are still breastfeeding after six months. If more than 20 percent are, it's a pretty good sign that the doctor is supportive of breastfeeding, in actions as well as words; more than 50 percent, it's an excellent sign. (She should also ask if any mothers with whom she works have continued to breastfeed after returning to work.) In general, she should avoid the doctors who say they are all for breastfeeding, yet have patients who are mostly bottle-fed.

The mother should be sure to ask how the doctor handles breastfeeding problems. Does she or he believe that babies should always be weaned if the mother develops a breast infection or sore nipples, or if the baby has thrush, diarrhea, or isn't gaining weight according to her expectations? These problems, among others, are better managed without weaning the baby.

The mother should ask other nursing mothers about their pediatricians or family doctors. If a mother is in touch with a lactation consultant, she can ask for the names of the doctors who refer patients to her. These women may lead a mother to a truly wonderful doctor who will support her not only in breastfeeding but as a mother, for many years to come.

BREAST CARE

Before the baby is born, the mother's body is preparing to feed the baby after birth. The mother's breasts are increasing in size as the blood flow to them increases and the milk-making structures within them develop. The areolae, the areas surrounding the nipples, are expanding and darkening. The glands in the areola begin to produce natural, antibacterial oils that will keep the nipples moist and protected during breastfeeding.

Halfway through their pregnancy, many mothers will be able to squeeze out small drops of honey-colored fluid, or colostrum, an extraordinary substance packed with nutrients that are perfect for newborns. This is the first food the baby will ever have. In fact, by the fifth or sixth month of pregnancy, a mother's breasts are fully capable of continuing to breastfeed her baby.

For the most part, therefore, nature is already preparing the mother's breasts for the job of nursing. The less the mother does, in most cases, the better. Soaps may wash off the natural oils produced by the glands in the areola. Creams may interfere with their antibacterial qualities. In the last three months of pregnancy, a mother may wish to stop using soap on her breasts at all. A simple rinse of clean water should suffice.

Some mothers may hear a lot about toughening up their nipples before the baby is born. While it is true that nature probably intended women's breasts to be more exposed to the sun, wind, and rain than breasts in developed countries usually are, sore nipples are usually the result of holding the baby in an incorrect position or of setting time limits while nursing.

Going braless to allow the gentle chafing of clothes against the nipples won't harm the mother, and may help prepare the nipples for nursing. It isn't absolutely necessary, however, even for fair-skinned women who are no more likely to have sore nipples than anyone else. Mothers should never rub their nipples with a brush or put rubbing alcohol or any other drying agents on them, for hard, dry skin is more likely to crack and more difficult to heal than soft, supple skin.

INVERTED NIPPLES

One exception to the rule of leaving well enough alone, however, is inverted nipples. Mothers should check around the sixth month of pregnancy to be sure that their nipples extend outward. Even if they have been somewhat inverted for most of a woman's life, pregnancy alone may extend them as the breasts swell and prepare for breastfeeding. Even if the nipples remain flat or inverted through pregnancy, the vigorous sucking of a healthy newborn may be all they require to function well. In rare cases, however, true inverted nipples need a little assistance to protrude enough so that the baby will be able to latch on and nurse.

If a woman is in doubt about the degree of inversion of her nipples, she can check them by gently squeezing just behind each with the thumb and forefinger. If one or both nipples do not protrude, but remain flat or even retract, a mother can take steps now to help them extend outward by the time the baby is born.

Plastic breast shells or cups are available from maternity stores, the La Leche League, and some lactation consultants. (Breast shells should be distinguished from nipple shields, which are not recommended.) Doughnut-shaped breast shells fit over the mother's nipples and exert a steady, gentle pressure on her areolae, loosening the adhesions beneath the nipples that are causing the inversion. A mother can wear shells comfortably under her bra from mid-pregnancy until birth. Wearing breast shells after birth, however, is not recommended as doing so may restrict her milk flow and lead to plugged ducts.

A simple exercise called the Hoffman technique may also loosen the adhesions that cause inversion. Several times a day, the mother should place her index fingers on her areolae and gently stretch them from side to side and up and down. Then she should carefully pull the nipple outward several times. Note that nipple stimulation can induce uterine contractions, however. If a mother has a history of premature labor, she should check with her doctor before doing these exercises or any activity that may stimulate her nipples.

CLOTHING AND OTHER PRODUCTS

Clothing specially made for nursing mothers is a convenience more than a necessity. Comfortable non-nursing bras that don't cinch or bind and that can easily pull down to expose the breast will work well enough. Mothers should be sure, however, to avoid any bra with an underwire, for they can lead to plugged ducts and breast infections.

Nursing bras are a lovely convenience if chosen carefully and well fitted. Available in maternity shops, lingerie departments, and through mail order catalogs, they come in a variety of styles. The mother should look for bras that can be both opened and closed with one hand, as she will usually need her other hand for her baby. One-hundred-percent cotton fabrics allow better air circulation, which will help keep the nipples dry and clean.

A mother should shop for a nursing bra about two weeks before her due date, because her breasts will be closest then to the size they will be during early nursing. A mother should plan on buying at least two, as bras do get wet from milk in the early days.

The leaking and spraying of the early days of nursing also make breast pads a popular convenience. Small, round pads of cotton fabric or absorbent paper, breast pads are available from maternity shops, mail order catalogs, and some drugstores. Some mothers love the more expensive fabric pads, particularly styles with a fitted dart sewn in. Other mothers find the disposable paper pads to be the easiest to use as they don't get lost in the piles of family laundry. Either way, pads made of synthetic materials or those with a layer of plastic between the fabric should be avoided, as these will keep the nipples moist and, perhaps, sore as well.

A mother may wish to invest in nightgowns that open in the front as well as daytime clothes (sweaters or shirts that lift from the waist) that allow easy and discreet access to the breasts. Attractive (and often pricey) nursing clothes are available through several mail order catalogs.

What other "equipment" does the breastfeeding mother require? If she is returning to work, or even if not, she eventually may wish to own a breast pump. Most lactation consultants, however, recommend waiting until after the baby is born and after breastfeeding is well established before purchasing or renting a breast pump. They would prefer that the mother focus on the baby and on nursing before worrying too much about learning to pump and giving a bottle to the baby. Nevertheless, if the time does come, a mother should plan to purchase or rent the best pump available—one with a sucking cycle of at least 45, but preferably 60, times per minute, to mimic the sucking of the baby. A high-quality pump will keep the milk supply strong, if she will be separated from the baby more than a few hours a day, and will help obtain the most milk in the least amount of time. Hospital-grade pumps have the fastest sucking cycles.

Bottles? Breastfed babies don't need bottles of formula, water, or even expressed breast milk. All they really need is their mother. If the baby will be drinking occasionally from a bottle down the road—because the mother is going back to work or because she wants to leave an expressed bottle of milk with a babysitter—she should wait until the third or fourth week to purchase one, which is the earliest a breastfed baby should be introduced to a rubber nipple.

Gale Pryor is a children's book editor and the author of *Working Mother, Nursing Mother: The Essential Guide to Breastfeeding and Staying Close to Your Baby After Returning to Work*. With her mother, Karen Pryor, she wrote *Nursing Your Baby*. She is also the mother of three boys, all of whom were breastfed through their toddler years while she worked full-time.

Breast milk comes naturally, but getting it into the baby may not. This chapter explores ways in which health professionals can help the new mother and the new baby get their act together and their lives together off to a good start.

Chapter 3
Getting Breastfeeding Started

The Critical First Few Days

Pamela K. Wiggins, I.B.C.L.C.

While a mother's body produces breast milk naturally, breastfeeding itself does not always come naturally to mothers and babies. It is often a learned art, and can require patience and perseverance during those critical first few days. New mothers often need—and should be offered—help at this important juncture in their relationship with their child. There are certain key points that will help: proper latching-on, correct positioning, and knowing when and how long to nurse will help ensure success.

IN THE HOSPITAL

It is very important to get off to a good start in the hospital, and it is not always easy. Medications given during labor may affect babies and make them too sleepy or too uninterested to nurse. Or the baby may, for one reason or another, have to stay in the central nursery, instead of rooming in with mom. Cesareans and other difficult deliveries are also factors that affect whether or not a mother feels up to breastfeeding. And well-meaning nurses often encourage mothers to rest while the nurses bottle-feed the baby. Whatever the reason, hospital routines often interfere with breastfeeding.

The sooner breastfeeding is begun, the better. Ideally, the baby will nurse within the first hour or so. This is the standard urged by the American Pediatrics Association. Babies are very alert during the first two hours and will be more likely to latch on well then than they will for the next twenty-four hours. The doctor or midwife should know that the mother wants to nurse soon after delivery.

Apgar scores and other measurements can wait a few minutes, as can baby's first bath.

Babies instinctively know how to breastfeed. When put near the breast, they will nuzzle, lick, root (bobbing their heads with open mouths, looking for the breast), and eventually find the nipple and latch on. A newborn baby, when placed on the mother's abdomen, can actually crawl to the breast and latch on with no outside help.

Rooming-in while in the hospital is best. It will definitely help both mother and baby get off to a good start. It enhances bonding and allows the mother to watch her baby for subtle signs that show her when the baby needs to nurse.

POSITIONING AND LATCH-ON

How the baby is held is very important. If he is not positioned just right, and latched on and breastfeeding effectively, it will interfere with milk production—which depends on milk being removed regularly. It doesn't matter which position a mother uses; latching-on is always the same. If a baby is correctly latched,

- he will have a good mouthful of breast in his mouth (so that his gums can compress the sinuses)
- his tongue will be covering the bottom gum
- his nose will be touching (or almost touching) the breast
- his chin will be tucked in close, so that his lower jaw is as far from the nipple as possible
- more of the areolae will be showing above the baby's top lip than at the bottom, and
- both lips will be flanged out.

There are several ways to position the baby. The most common way is called the cradle hold.

- The mother should sit in a comfortable chair or in a sitting position in bed. Extra pillows will help support the baby.
- The baby's head should be on the mother's forearm with his face directly facing the breast. The baby's whole body should be facing the mother's body. The baby's back should be supported by the mother's arm and his bottom held up by her hand. The baby's whole body must be level with her breast and she shouldn't lean forward. (Pillows in her lap will help support the baby.) The mother's other hand should support the breast (near the areola) in the C-hold (thumb above and four fingers underneath.)

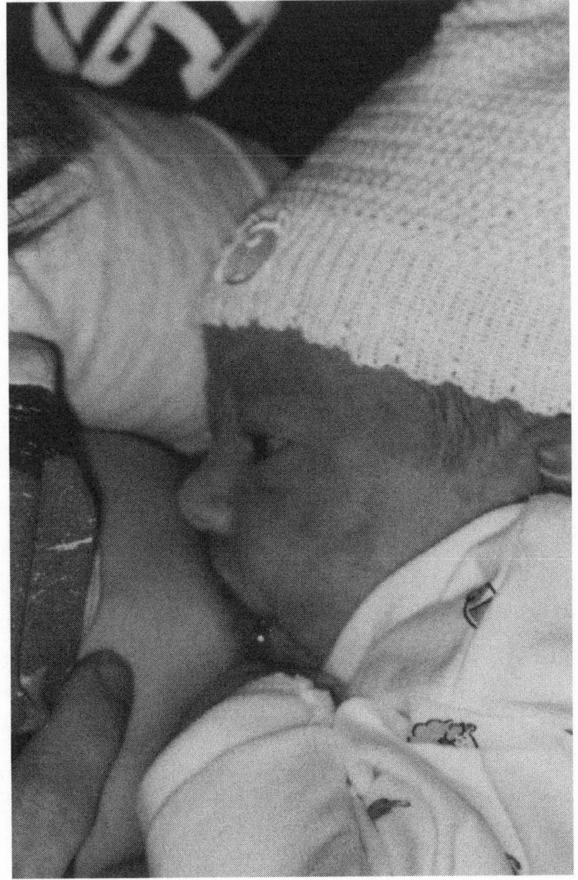

In latching on, the baby will have a good mouthful of breast, so that his gums can compress the sinuses and his tongue will be covering the bottom gum. His nose will almost be touching the breast. No matter what position the mother is in, the latch-on is always the same.

A mother who has had a cesarean can still nurse in the cradle-hold position. She may need help getting propped up and/or help arranging extra pillows that will protect the incision.

- Many C-section mothers are comfortable using the "lying down" position. The nurse should help the mother turn over onto her side so the baby can lie facing the breast.
- Other C-section mothers prefer the "football hold." It is also a good way to nurse twins at the same time.
- Again, the mother should sit in a comfortable chair or be propped up in bed. Pillows under each arm will help. The baby is held on her arm with his feet toward her back. The baby's neck and shoulders should be supported by his mother's hand.

There is one other position to be familiar with. It is called the "across the lap hold." In this position the baby is held across the lap, as in the cradle hold, but the baby's neck and shoulders are supported by the mother's hand (instead of her forearm). The other hand supports her breast (in the C-hold). The baby should still be facing the mother. It is a little more difficult to keep the baby close enough to the breast for successful nursing in this position.

Always, breastfeeding success depends on proper latching on, no matter what position is used.

COLOSTRUM

Even though a mother begins breastfeeding right after birth, she won't produce breast milk right away. The first few days after the birth, the breasts produce a power-packed substance called colostrum, which is usually yellow-colored or clear. It is very rich in proteins and helps protect the baby from illness. Colostrum gradually turns to "white milk" in two to four days.

Colostrum is very important to the baby. Although some cultures believe colostrum to be harmful, nothing could be further from the truth. It is liquid gold. Newborns need colostrum, not only for the valuable nutrients and immunities it provides, but to help prevent jaundice. Colostrum acts as a laxative and helps move meconium along, that is, the waste built up in utero. Meconium is loaded with bilirubin, the extra red blood cells babies need in utero). Bilirubin is broken down and eliminated during the early weeks of life. If not passed quickly, the bilirubin will be reabsorbed and the baby will become jaundiced. (Other theories about jaundice in babies are mentioned elsewhere.)

ENGORGEMENT

On the day the milk does "come in," some women will experience engorgement (breast swelling). Often, breastfeeding from birth will help to prevent this. Engorgement occurs most often when the baby hasn't nursed frequently enough and milk hasn't been removed regularly.

If the breasts do swell and are tender, the mother should nurse often and use a breast pump or hand express between feedings, if necessary. Massaging her breasts with warm, wet cloths or standing in a warm shower will also help. And putting ice packs on the breasts after feedings or pumping will help reduce swelling.

Sometimes a breast is so swollen that the nipple "flattens out" and the baby can't latch on. If this happens, the mother must express or pump out a little milk before beginning to nurse. With proper management, engorgement will only last one or two days.

HOW OFTEN TO NURSE

Babies need to be nursed often during the first few days. In fact, they need to nurse on demand—unless they don't "demand" to nurse frequently enough. Babies who are too sleepy or too medicated from labor often don't care whether they eat or not, so the mother must be diligent. She must wake her infant and nurse him at least every two to three hours in the first day or two.

After the first few days, the baby can generally be fed on demand. The mother will learn to recognize her baby's hunger signals. He will start to fuss, squirm, chew his fists, and/or root. Mothers should be urged to recognize their baby's signals and feed the baby when needed. There is no need to wait until the baby cries; a crying baby may, in fact, be too upset to nurse. Mothers should not be afraid of spoiling a baby. Experts agree that you can't spoil a newborn.

Sometimes breastfeeding mothers compare their baby's schedule to a bottle baby's. However, breast milk is digested much faster than formula, so breastfed babies must be fed more often. Putting them on a schedule just won't work for the first few weeks. As time goes by, when their stomachs can hold more, and they get more efficient at getting milk, babies will get into a routine of feeding about every three hours.

HOW LONG TO NURSE

There are two kinds of milk: foremilk and hindmilk. Foremilk is thin and watery and is released at the beginning of the feed. Hindmilk is higher in fat and calories and comes down later in a feeding. The baby knows exactly how much foremilk and hindmilk he needs, so letting him decide how long to nurse on each breast is best. Ideally, he will nurse until he comes off the first breast on his own. It will take at least fifteen minutes, possibly more. If he is fully satisfied, there is no need to try to put him on the second breast. If he seems to want more, then he should be nursed on the other side. Some mothers find it easier to use only one breast per feeding. It takes about thirty minutes and babies get more of the high-fat creamy milk.

SUPPLEMENTARY BOTTLES OF FORMULA OR WATER

Well-intentioned friends may suggest to a mother that she introduce some formula while the child is still very young. They may give her all sorts of justification for this, such as, "Your baby needs to get used to a rubber nipple or you will never be able to go anywhere without him," or "Your baby should get used to the taste of formula," or "The father should be able to feed him," and so forth. But mothers shouldn't be tempted to give the baby a bottle.

Bottle-feeding is quite different from sucking at the mother's breast, and many babies have become confused or prefer the bottle after only one or two feedings. They actually seem to forget how to breastfeed. It takes a little more effort for the baby to nurse, since he has to move both his jaws and his tongue a certain way to get milk. With a bottle, all he has to do is create a suction and then swallow. Nipple-confused babies can often be retaught to breastfeed with the help of a lactation consultant. Water is unnecessary for a completely breastfed baby, even in hot climates.

AFTER-PAINS

In the first few hours or days of nursing the mother may feel the uterus contracting (cramping) when the baby nurses. This means the baby is latched on correctly and the uterus is getting back to normal. After-pains soon go away. If the after-pains are extremely painful, the mother should tell the nurse and take a painkiller about a half hour before nursing.

A FINAL WORD OF ADVICE

Breastfeeding isn't always easy in the first few days. Giving birth is a major event and it takes a while for mother and baby to settle into a nice rhythm. Ideally, the mother will have help with housework and family meals while recuperating, so she will be able to concentrate on taking care of her baby.

The keys to successful breastfeeding are correct latching on, proper positioning, and nursing the baby when he needs to nurse. Once these things are right, everything else will fall into place. Breastfeeding will become easy for mother and baby, and both will benefit greatly from it.

Pamela Wiggins, I.B.C.L.C., is an International Board Certified Lactation Consultant with over twenty years' experience. She teaches breastfeeding classes for expectant parents and gives in-service training to nurses in Franklin, Virginia. She is the author of *Breastfeeding: A Mother's Gift and Why Should I Nurse My Baby,* a guide used by hospitals and health departments worldwide. The guide has sold over 400,000 copies and has been translated into four languages.

The longer a baby breastfeeds, the better, and this thorough discussion explains why. The chapter also includes a section on traditional times to begin weaning with traditional reasons for them, and explains alternative timing with sound, objective reasoning.

Chapter 4
Breastfeeding After Six Months

Pamela Morrison, I.B.C.L.C.

Breastfeeding a not-so-tiny baby into toddlerhood and beyond is not only easy and convenient, it can be one of life's richest experiences. As the months pass by, the mother who realizes with growing pride and confidence that her body can both nourish and nurture her baby, and that he thrives on her milk and her mothering, is coasting on the downhill run. So why stop?

If only it were that simple. How long a baby should continue to breastfeed is perhaps one of the most emotion-laden aspects of baby care in every culture and society. Most people, regardless of population group or background, feel very strongly about the subject. Every culture has long-standing traditions and laws governing how breastfeeding should take place, and when it should stop. Myth-information abounds. Although a mother instinctively knows that she is the expert on her own baby, she finds herself the recipient of advice and admonitions from family members, friends, health providers, and even total strangers who would not dream of criticizing her choice of hairstyle or the management of her household, but will have no hesitation at all in telling her how she should bring up her child!

MAKING AN INFORMED CHOICE

The facts of the matter are that the longer a child breastfeeds, the better the health outcome. Up-to-date infant feeding guidelines developed by UNICEF, the World Health Organization, and other expert bodies recommend that all babies—including those living in First World countries—should receive exclusive breastfeeding for the first four to six months of life, followed by the gradual introduction of nutritious, home-prepared weaning foods, along with continued partial

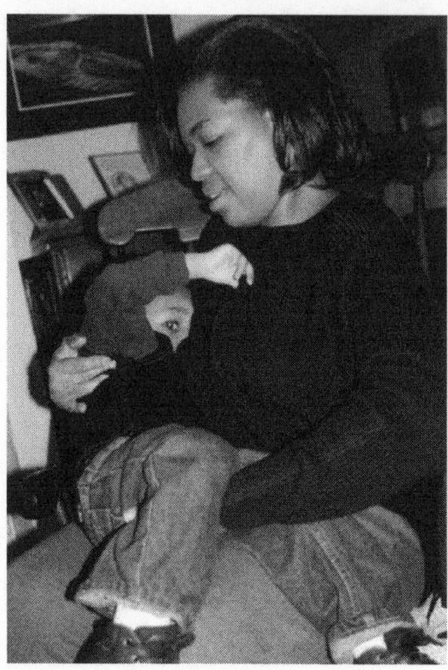

An older child—say, four to seven years of age—may seek out the comfort of his mother's breast when he is lonely, bored, sick, hurt, or simply being fractious. Nursing such a child may calm him, and he will often go back to playing or studying or whatever after a few minutes' solace.

breastfeeding for up to two years or beyond. In addition, a recent American Academy of Pediatrics statement indicates that twelve months should be the minimum duration of breastfeeding and does not establish any upper limit.

A full fifty percent of the world's children are still breastfeeding by their second birthday. Most of them continue for two to four years. Anthropological data suggests that in order to achieve optimal physical health, cognitive development, and emotional stability, breastfeeding should continue for two-and-a-half to seven years. In other words, with respect to breastfeeding, any is better than none, and more is better.

GOOD NUTRITION

The mother of an older baby can be assured that the quality of her milk remains excellent for her baby for as long as she cares to provide it. The practice of breastfeeding beyond six, twelve, and twenty-four months has often been neglected in research and nutritional studies, yet breast milk still provides the most important source of good-quality protein, vitamins A and C, calcium, and the long chain polyunsaturated fatty acids essential to normal brain development that are unobtainable from any other source.

One group of researchers found that breast-milk protein and lipid composition remained constant over twenty-three months of lactation. Further research showed that a baby seven to eighteen months old could receive fifty percent of his calories from breast milk, and that even from nineteen to thirty-six months he could still obtain more than ten percent. With 500 milliliters of breast milk per day, fifty percent of the daily requirement of absorbed iron and ninety-five percent of the vitamin C can be provided.

The quantity of breast milk produced at any stage of lactation is consumer-driven. According to Australian studies, the rate and quantity of breast milk synthesis is determined by how frequently and how efficiently the breasts are drained. Thus, the mother of an older baby who wishes to keep up her breast milk supply should continue to allow her child unlimited access to the breast.

PROTECTION FROM DISEASE

During the breastfeeding period there exists a mother–child bond that is not only emotional but also immunological. The young child's immune system may not be fully mature until he reaches six to seven years of age, and the older mobile baby is especially vulnerable because he is generally exposed to a variety of infections. Research shows that the mother's immune system can create a buffer against the outside world by manufacturing specific antibodies to specific infections, as the need arises, to be passed to the baby in her milk.

Babies of all ages who are still breastfed experience lower rates of disease. Furthermore, when the older breastfed baby does become sick, the duration of the illness is reduced and its severity is decreased. Only breastfeeding can protect babies against the gastroenteritis and respiratory infections for which no immunizations are yet available. Research indicates that as natural weaning progresses during the second year of life, and as the volume of milk decreases, so the level of the antibodies rises. Some immune components, such as lysozyme and lactoferrin, reach their highest levels in breast milk during the second year of breastfeeding, and one study has showed that levels of IgA and IgG at twenty months reached levels found in milk produced during the second week of postpartum.

Because of lack of research on the health implications for children breastfed for longer than two years, there is no basis for any recommendation, medical or otherwise, that breastfeeding should end at any particular time.

The full protective effects of extended breastfeeding are still being established as the results of epidemiological studies are published, but all the studies conducted to date show that the longer the duration of breastfeeding—up to twenty-four months—the better the health outcome, and there is no age at which mother's milk in any amount, no matter how small, ceases to be beneficial.

The supreme adaptability of the human female breast is particularly evident during times of sickness. The mother of an ill baby who seems to have lost his appetite for other foods will find that as she comforts him by more frequent nursing, she achieves the effect of increasing her breast milk supply to match his needs for fluids and nutrition. Research indicates that children who are still breastfeeding have a smaller drop in energy intakes during illness. When diarrhea occurs, breastfeeding is an essential element in recovery. Researchers have verified that approximately six hundred milliliters of breast milk per day will preclude oral rehydration therapy, and if a sick child can take anything at all by mouth, it should be breast milk. Hospitalized children need their mothers and, if encouraged to breastfeed on demand day and night, will stimulate ample milk secretion with frequent suckling.

THE IDEAL MOTHERING TOOL

The mother who elects to follow the baby's lead and continues to place no limits on breastfeeding as her baby grows older takes advantage of the most effective mothering tool yet invented: her ability, through breastfeeding, to keep her child happy and healthy at the same time. It may seem, in practical terms, that the comfort aspects of nursing take precedence over the nutritional benefits of breastfeeding. It is clearly easier and more emotionally satisfying, as well as more convenient and cost-effective, for a mother to continue breastfeeding an older child rather than to wean him. Yet the nutritional, immunological, and comfort aspects of breastfeeding are inseparably intertwined and each has been shown to be vital to the well-being of the older nursling.

The older baby-child may seek out the solace and comfort of the breast whenever he is tired, lonely, bored, sick, or hurt. Nursing mothers of older babies are aware of the convenience of "breast-propping" whenever they want to sit and read a book, chat with their husbands, talk on the phone, or take a well-earned rest. A few minutes spent nursing a fractious, out-of-control two-year-old may seem to calm him and to simultaneously charge up his batteries, so that he will slide off his mother's lap to explore more of his exciting new world, seeming better able to take its frustrations in his stride.

Nursing can take away the pain of a bumped head or a scraped knee, as well as staunch the bleeding of a mouth injury, and serves to comfort both anxious mother and hurt toddler.

OVER-DEPENDENCE VERSUS SELF-CONFIDENCE

It needs to be acknowledged that human children mature slowly and that they are dependent for a long period. The mother need not be afraid to "baby the baby" who may wish to nurse more often if he is developing a cold or other infection, or if he is developing very fast in another area such as motor, verbal, or social skills. Nursing on demand is obviously appropriate in these circumstances, and the mother may be aware that her baby's personal crisis is over when he no longer needs to nurse so often.

Concerns about over-dependence and clinginess in an older nursing child are frequently cited as reasons for weaning. However, a study involving women who elected to pursue child-led weaning showed that these mothers perceived their still-nursing toddlers to be more self-confident and outgoing than children who were weaned earlier. The older nursing child has the solace of his mother's welcoming arms and breast to return to whenever the world becomes too overwhelming or too painful for him to handle. Researchers have also found that test scores of children on scales of cognitive and motor development increase in proportion to the duration of breastfeeding, leading to increased self-confidence on the part of the child. One scientific researcher concludes, "Overwhelming evidence shows that meeting the dependency needs of children during the first few years of life results in independent, self-sufficient, physically and emotionally healthy children."

NIGHTTIME NEEDS

Like all mammal young who are immature and thus vulnerable, the majority of the world's babies sleep with their mothers and wake often in the night to breastfeed. In industrialized countries, however, it is often believed that babies should "sleep through the night" alone in their own rooms, and give up night feedings at a particular age.

These beliefs can create great distress when the baby refuses to comply with the parents' efforts to mold him to the cultural norm. Recent research on co-sleeping shows that waking in the night is normal and provides a safety mechanism for the baby against the risk of Sudden Infant Death Syndrome. Babies who sleep alone are more at risk than babies who sleep in close proximity to their mothers, and the mother who elects to respond to her older baby's nighttime needs continues to protect him, not spoil him.

Many toddlers are fussy eaters, but nighttime nursers, who may take as much as 75 percent of their breast milk during the hours of darkness, are apt to be better nourished than their non-nursing counterparts. In practical terms, breastfeeding at night makes life easier for the mother. Toddlers can be nursed to sleep in a mere five minutes at the end of a busy day and will often ask to go to bed, because they know that bedtime is a delicious, snuggly time as they drift off to sleep at the breast in mother's arms. The nursing mother who sleeps in close proximity to her baby has an easy and ever available means of calming and comforting a wakeful child back to sleep, frequently without fully awakening herself. Mothers of children who were particularly wakeful toddlers consistently report higher-than-average academic performance once these children start school.

BREASTFEEDING IN PUBLIC

Cultural differences about breastfeeding in front of others vary widely depending on which society is being observed. In Africa the sight of a mother breastfeeding her baby in public is unremarkable. Mothers and babies nurse at busy street intersections, outside banks and supermarkets, and on the bus. African mothers whose babies cry in public receive the strong message from anyone in the vicinity to offer the breast and so keep them quiet.

Women who live in places where breastfeeding is not the cultural norm—and particularly in societies where the primary function of the female breast is seen to be sexual—have been criticized, harassed, and even prosecuted for breastfeeding in public. Mothers have developed various coping strategies, including "closet nursing," where breastfeeding takes place only in the privacy of their own homes, and encouraging older nursing children to use code words for nursing such as "Nummies" or "Bee-boo" in order to save embarrassment. In recent years many countries and states have passed legislation to prevent harassment of nursing mothers so that more realistic attitudes now prevail. This achievement is largely due to mothers who have been willing to withstand public criticism—thereby modeling normal, natural nursing for other women—and to lobby for laws that are more "baby-friendly."

WHAT'S IN IT FOR MOM?

Notwithstanding the culturally determined early weaning practices prevalent in Western industrialized societies, accusations that long-term breastfeeding is abnormal or serves only to enhance the mother's own emotional satisfaction have not been backed by research. There are also health benefits for the mother who breastfeeds her child into toddlerhood and beyond. Lactation has been called the biological continuum of pregnancy. Mothers can supply breast milk to their children for long periods without suffering nutritionally themselves. The release of prolactin (often called "nature's tranquilizer"), which occurs during nursing, can help the mother maintain an emotionally even keel in the hectic and challenging role as the mother of a toddler, and can delay ovulation and menstruation—sometimes for up to two years—providing a natural form of child-spacing. As milk is slowly replaced by weaning foods, the breasts gradually involute to their pre-pregnant state, and research confirms that long-term lactation can lead to a reduced risk of pre- and post-menopausal breast cancer.

Breastfeeding is designed to be a pleasurable experience for the mother as well as the child. A woman who is "in touch" with her child many times a day is able to communicate with him more effectively than if he were already weaned. Thus, her self-esteem is enhanced, as time goes on, by knowing that her mothering achieves such excellent results.

CULTURE VERSUS REALITY

In societies where breastfeeding an older baby is seen to be unusual, criticism of mothers who continue to nurse increases in direct proportion to the age of the child. A mother may receive both subtle and overt messages from books, magazines, and her peers, which range from encouragement to "get back to normal" (implying that pregnancy and lactation are abnormal conditions for women) to outright disgust at the sight of a child big enough to be running around "still doing that."

Unexpected pressure may come from the mother's older female relatives or advisors who themselves may have experienced little of the joy of breastfeeding, due to the paucity of assistance in breastfeeding a generation or two ago. A mother may be urged to put as much distance between herself and her baby as possible; to avoid picking him up every time he cries; to teach him self-calming techniques; to use mother-substitutes such as swings and pacifiers; to sleep apart from him; and above all not to breastfeed him every time he asks for it. The focus is frequently on the mother, rather than on a realistic acceptance of the needs of the more vulnerable baby. Furthermore, it is often implied that her relationship with the baby's father should take precedence over her baby's continued need for her milk and that her presence and even her breasts are her husband's "property."

In less affluent societies such practices would seriously compromise child survival. It is small wonder, then, that the conscientious First World mother experiences feelings of sadness and anger that may border on grief or depression if she weans her baby prematurely. The awareness that the length of the nursing relationship is determined by society, rather than by the natural laws governing survival of the species, may help a mother to realize that she is the one left "holding the baby" and it is she alone who will bear the main responsibility for her child's continued health and happiness. With an acknowledgment that the duration of breastfeeding will have a profound impact on her baby/child's emotional, intellectual, and physical well-being for the rest of his life, the very best thing a mother can do is to let Nature take its course and leave the decision about how long to breastfeed up to the baby.

MARKERS FOR WEANING: MYTH VERSUS REALITY

Baby's first birthday: Anthropological and medical research show the ideal duration of breastfeeding to be two-and-a-half to seven years.

When baby has teeth: Which teeth? Lower incisors, two-year-old molars, adult teeth? Weaning for other primates occurs as adult teeth develop. Development of teeth in the human baby does not preclude breastfeeding. Potential biting can be discouraged.

When baby starts walking: The normal interval for learning to walk in human babies is eight to eighteen months, whereas other mammals can walk at birth. There is no medical reason for weaning when baby walks.

When baby starts talking: Babies may say their first word at seven to eight months. A mother can encourage a "code word" for breastfeeding if she is embarrassed by a verbal child asking to nurse in public. No medical/health benefit to weaning at this point.

When baby develops sufficient manual dexterity to undo mother's clothing: Developmental skills are no research-based reason for weaning.

Baby starting playgroup/preschool: Benefits of continued breastfeeding include increased protection from infection as the child mixes with other children.

Separation from baby overnight: African belief that milk "spoils." Not a reason for weaning. Mother can express her milk during separation to maintain breast comfort—reducing risk of mastitis, and maintaining her breast milk supply—and resume nursing on her return.

New pregnancy: Industrialized countries may believe that continued breastfeeding endangers the health of the mother or fetus. African cultures may believe that milk turns "poisonous" and child nursing will be harmed. Neither belief supported by research; breastfeeding can continue.

Sudden breast refusal by the baby: Natural weaning is always gradual. Sudden refusal is called a "nursing strike" and can be resolved. Breastfeeding should continue.

Baby not eating enough "real food": Older babies may refuse other foods if sick or in cases of food sensitivity. Breastfeeding should be increased to make up extra caloric needs. Weaning can lead to malnutrition, inadequate weight gain or growth, or both.

For baby's own good: Closer examination of this statement always reveals perceived benefits for the mother, such as more time for herself/sleep/social activities/time with husband.

BREASTFEEDING DURING SPECIAL SITUATIONS

Working

Returning to work or school does not preclude continued nursing. It is possible for the mother to pump or manually express her milk to maintain continued milk production during separations. Expressed breast milk can be stored and fed to the baby during her absence and nursing can continue at night and over the weekends. This requires careful planning, but has important advantages to mother and baby, including reduced episodes of infection and therefore lower rates of absenteeism from work.

Medications

Continued breastfeeding is easier and safer than weaning when a mother requires medication or if she is sick or hospitalized. The large majority of prescribed drugs and diagnostic tests are compatible with breastfeeding. If not, the mother should discuss the possibility of alternatives with her doctor or seek a second opinion. Health complications can occur with abrupt weaning, and the risks to the baby from not breastfeeding are nearly always greater than any potential risk from the small quantity of a drug ingested via breast milk. See chapter 18, "Medications and the Breastfeeding Mother," and chapter 20, "When Not to Breastfeed."

Nursing Strikes

Sudden breast refusal on the part of an older baby or child should not be mistaken for weaning, which is always a very gradual process. Older babies whose tolerance level has been stretched too far may "go on strike." A medical checkup is always appropriate in cases of sudden breast refusal to rule out a baby's ear or other infections. A persistent mother can usually coax a striking baby back to the breast by staying calm, not forcing him, and employing all the persuasive strategies at her disposal. In the meantime, the mother can express or pump her milk to keep up her supply, and can seek help from a breastfeeding specialist if the baby does not resume nursing within a couple of days.

Other Foods

An older baby may want to nurse as often as a newborn, but for shorter times. Once the baby begins taking weaning foods, it is helpful to offer the breast first and in between meals and add other foods as desired. Early weaning can be minimized by offering the baby other drinks in a cup, by making weaning foods less liquid, and by avoiding giving the baby sweet drinks in a bottle, so that most of his fluids and all of his needs for breastfeeding are met at the breast.

Erratic Nursing

Older children can be very erratic in their nursing patterns, nursing many times one day and hardly at all the next. To avoid overfull breasts during long intervals between breastfeeds, the mother may want to remind her older nursling to breastfeed. Failing his cooperation, she should pump or express her milk and treat any symptoms of a plugged duct or mastitis promptly and aggressively.

Pummeling or Pinching

Older babies may want a quick reward during breastfeeding and may become very adept at pushing, pinching, and kneading the breast (like kittens) or twiddling the other nipple to stimulate a faster flow of milk. If the mother objects to any of these behaviors she can, of course, let her baby know and use breast compression to stimulate a faster letdown of breast milk.

Biting

If biting occurs, the baby needs to be told kindly, but firmly, that it is not permitted. The first time it happens, the mother can set the baby on the floor, resume nursing if he cries, but set him on the floor immediately if he bites again. Offer acceptable alternatives to bite on, such as hard, cold, or chewy objects. Babies learn very quickly that biting the breast is not appropriate.

Sexual Implications

An older nursing child may demonstrate the difference between sensuality and sexuality. There is no evidence to support the contention that continued breastfeeding of either an older girl baby or a boy baby will interfere with that child's sexual orientation in adulthood. To the baby, breastfeeding is a means of obtaining food, comfort, and security from the person he loves most in the world, nothing more. It is simply not possible to force an older child to nurse past the time that he no longer needs to breastfeed.

Superimposed Pregnancy

Although many women choose to wean the older nursling, there is no physical or medical reason why breastfeeding cannot continue during a new pregnancy. Although there may be cultural taboos in some societies about breastfeeding during a subsequent pregnancy, mothers need to be reassured that continued nursing will not harm the baby *in utero*, the older nursling, or the mother herself. Many mothers have elected to breastfeed an older sibling and a younger baby at the same time. This is called "tandem nursing."

METHODS TO FACILITATE A LONGER NURSING COURSE

The comfort aspects of nursing may frequently be undervalued by society in general, yet this may be the main motivation for the older nursling to continue breastfeeding.

Healthcare providers who were assisting mothers of already weaned, malnourished children to re-lactate at Harare Hospital in Zimbabwe found that one- to two-year-olds who liked to touch the mother's skin, often sliding a small hand down the mother's dress to reach the breasts, were the ones most likely to resume nursing—thereby ensuring their own recovery. Mothers and babies whose relationship was characterized by less warmth and more distance were less likely to be successful in re-lactation efforts, regardless of the quantity of milk being produced.

Thus, mothers who wish to take advantage of a longer nursing period can take measures that are likely to enhance the whole mother-baby relationship:

1. Holding and carrying the baby often
2. Sleeping with the baby at night
3. Responding promptly to his requests to breastfeed
4. Giving him focused attention during nursing times
5. Nursing in a quiet spot without too many distractions
6. As far as possible, making nursing into a deliciously special mom-and-baby time

---

Pamela Morrison, I.B.C.L.C., is a former La Leche League Leader and has worked as a Lactation Consultant in private practice in Harare, Zimbabwe, since 1991. She has served on the ILCA Code committee and is a national facilitator, assessor, and member of the Zimbabwe Baby-Friendly Hospital Initiative task force.

One of the many ways in which breastfeeding is best for the baby—and one that is often overlooked—is that it helps the mouth, teeth, and swallowing reflex of the child to develop properly. Although orthodontia in later life can sometimes alleviate the problems caused by bottle-feeding and pacifier use, this chapter discusses how to avoid the problems entirely.

Chapter 5
Breastfeeding for Proper Occlusion

Into the Mouths of Babes

Ros Escott, B. App. Sc., I.B.C.L.C.

Breast or bottle? You've undoubtedly heard that "breast is best," that breast milk has many advantages over infant formula.

But are you also aware that feeding from the breast, rather than from an artificial nipple on a bottle, helps the mouth and jaws to develop properly, laying the foundation for learning the correct ways to chew, swallow, breathe, and speak? Prolonged use of a bottle nipple or pacifier can affect the development of the baby's mouth, teeth, swallowing, and airways, and the consequences can persist into childhood, adolescence, and adulthood.

Not every baby who is bottle-fed or uses a pacifier will have problems in any or all of these areas. However, our ancestors who were fully breastfed had well-formed mouths and teeth. Anthropologists are unable to find the bony malformations we consider associated with bottle-feeding. Unnatural objects in the mouth mean a greater risk of problems occurring, now or later. Pacifier use is believed to increase middle-ear infections in young children by 25%, while bottle-feeding practices are responsible for 95% of severe tooth decay in young children.

We also know that babies who are bottle-fed are nearly twice as likely to develop malocclusion—poor alignment of the teeth, which often requires orthodontic treatment. The risk for malocclusion may depend on the extent of artificial nipple use. For example, the greatest risk may be bottle plus pacifier, introduced early and used day and night for two or more years. Variations in sucking technique and vigor of the individual infant may be contributing factors to differences in how particular babies are affected.

Before a mother puts any unnatural object such as a feeding bottle or pacifier into her baby's mouth, she should take into account that the bones of the face and mouth are quite soft in infancy and easily pushed out of shape by abnormal pressures in the mouth, or pulled out of shape by early overdevelopment of the wrong sets of muscles. Breastfeeding helps the mouth and face develop as nature intended.

Breast tissue is relatively soft and pliable, so it conforms to the unique shape of the baby's mouth, filling all the available space and exerting a gentle, evenly distributed pressure. In contrast, artificial nipples on bottles are stiffer than the breast and have a predetermined shape so the baby's mouth and tongue have to adapt to that shape. With every suck, the nipple is pushed by the tongue against the soft bones of the roof of the mouth and if the nipple is firm it can gradually force the bone up into a high, narrow arch.

Feeding is a baby's first workout. The rhythmic sucking movements of the mouth are repeated hundreds of times at each feeding, thousands of time each day. If such frequent repetition is continued over a long period, even small differences in feeding technique can have an exaggerated effect on the developing mouth. There are distinct differences between the way a baby feeds from the breast and the way the baby feeds from the bottle. The tongue is in a different position, different groups of muscles are used, and the baby's swallow reflex is different.

FEEDING FROM A BREAST

To breastfeed, the baby's mouth opens wide to take in a good mouthful of breast. The nipple is drawn to the back of the mouth, and the tongue cups around the elongated breast tissue and nipple. The breast is milked not by suction, but by a circular movement of the jaw (down, out, up, in) and a ripple-like movement of the muscles in the center of the tongue, front to back. This gently presses the breast tissue against the roof of the mouth and squeezes the milk out.

FEEDING FROM A BOTTLE NIPPLE

Artificial nipples are preformed, so once they are inserted or drawn into the mouth, no muscular action is required by the tongue to hold the nipple in place or to elongate it. In fact the tongue tends to hump at the back, probably to control milk flow into the throat. Milk is obtained using suction generated by the cheeks, and an up–down motion of the jaw and tongue. This is vigorous exercise, but it develops the wrong muscles. When these muscles pull on the soft bones, they can slowly change the shape of the mouth, making it narrower with less space for the teeth and tongue.

SWALLOWING

Breast milk comes from 15 to 20 tiny duct openings on the face of the nipple. The artificial nipple usually has only one hole or slit, so the milk tends to gush if the hole is large, or come out in a thin, hard stream if the hole is small. The most effective way for the baby to control this flow, and coordinate breathing and swallowing, is to feed with the bottle nipple closer to the front of the mouth and the tongue humped up to control the flow. As the muscles develop to support this type of action, they can set up a habit called "tongue thrust swallow." This means that the tongue unnaturally thrusts forward against the front teeth during swallowing, eventually pushing them out or up so they don't meet properly with the lower teeth and cause problems with biting and chewing.

Dentists with an interest in this field see this type of swallowing more commonly in children who were bottle-fed, and it sometimes can persist into adult life.

During a normal adult swallow, the tongue tip is raised to sit behind the upper front teeth, with the sides of the tongue curving up to form a seal with the roof of the mouth. Lip closure is not necessary. The food, drink, or saliva is organized into the central channel of the tongue before being moved to the throat by a movement that passes along the tongue, from front to back.

In tongue-thrust swallowing, the tongue tip presses against or between the front teeth. To help form a seal, the lips close and the cheeks may be sucked in slightly. If the tongue cannot organize the food efficiently into a central channel, it is difficult to move it back to the throat. To help with swallowing, people who use this method of swallowing may need to sip water throughout their meals.

We swallow hundreds of times each day, about 73,000 times each year. It is not difficult to appreciate that an unnatural force of the tongue against the front teeth, repeated so frequently, will eventually push the teeth out of alignment.

> *My teeth were straightened in my teens but have since relapsed, so now I've got braces again in my thirties. This time I'm doing exercises to correct my tongue thrust. My kids laugh at me when I do things like try to swallow water while holding a raisin above my teeth with the tip of my tongue. They can do it easily, but then they were breastfed.*
>
> Jill, bottle-fed from one month of age, mother of three

A study of 845 children under age three in day care centers found that pacifier use was associated with a 25% increase in attacks of middle-ear infection. An abnormal tongue position during swallowing can interfere with the eustachian tubes, which drain fluid from the ear to the throat. A buildup of fluid in the ears can lead to infection.

MALOCCLUSION

All babies are born with the upper and lower gums out of alignment, but the muscular movements of breastfeeding stimulate the lower jaw to develop so that it grows into the correct position. When a baby is bottle-fed, the underdeveloped lower jaw may persist, or may develop incorrectly, so that the upper and lower teeth can't meet properly. This is called malocclusion, and its correction is the most common reason for orthodontic treatment.

A study of over 9,500 children aged 3 to 17 found that children who were bottle-fed were nearly twice as likely to have malocclusion as children who were breastfed. They also found that the longer the child was breastfed, the lower the risk. Another study found that children who had used orthodontic pacifiers had a greater tendency to have an overdeveloped lower jaw, whereas users of conventional pacifiers had higher rates of open bite, a gap between the upper and lower front teeth when the back teeth are in contact.

AIRWAYS

The soft bones forming the roof of the mouth can be pushed up and molded by the repeated pressure of a firm bottle nipple or pacifier. When this happens, the floor of the nasal chamber is also pushed up. This decreases the space of the nasal airway, and can make it more difficult to breathe through the nose. This is made worse if the child also has allergies, and may lead to mouth breathing, poor sleep quality, snoring, and frequent upper respiratory tract infections.

TEETH

In 95% of cases baby bottle tooth decay—severe decay in the primary teeth of very young children—has been found to be caused by bottle-feeding practices, which prolong the time the teeth are in contact with the bottle contents, as this contact provides a steady source of food for the bacteria that cause tooth decay.

When a child is breastfed, antibacterial and other properties in breast milk protect the teeth from sugar (lactose) in the milk. Our ancestors were breastfed for several years, and anthropologists have found that there was almost no evidence of tooth decay in their primary teeth. But with all the processed foods in our modern diet, this protection is not 100% after other food and drink are introduced. Unfortunately, dental decay does occur before the age of two in some long-term breastfed children.

EARLY TOOTH DECAY

Dr. Harry Torney, an Irish dentist, studied children who had been breastfed for at least two years, including a group who had signs of early dental decay. He found no relationship between the age of weaning and the frequency of breastfeeding during the day or night. However, the children with decay appeared to have defects in the enamel of their primary teeth, which had formed before birth. He found that, during pregnancy, their mothers were more likely to have suffered stress, had an illness with high fever, taken antibiotics, or had a lower intake of calcium. He concluded that it was not solely the breastfeeding that caused decay, but that the children were born with susceptible teeth.

Weaning is not necessary if early tooth decay is detected, but dental hygiene measures should be thoroughly addressed. Wiping the teeth with a soft cloth after night feeds may be necessary. Other feeding habits and the rest of the diet should also be checked.

> *When Tom was nearly two years old, and still breastfed, I noticed he had areas of decay on his front teeth, near the gumline. The dentist asked me lots of questions and laid the blame on the cup of diluted juice I was giving him*

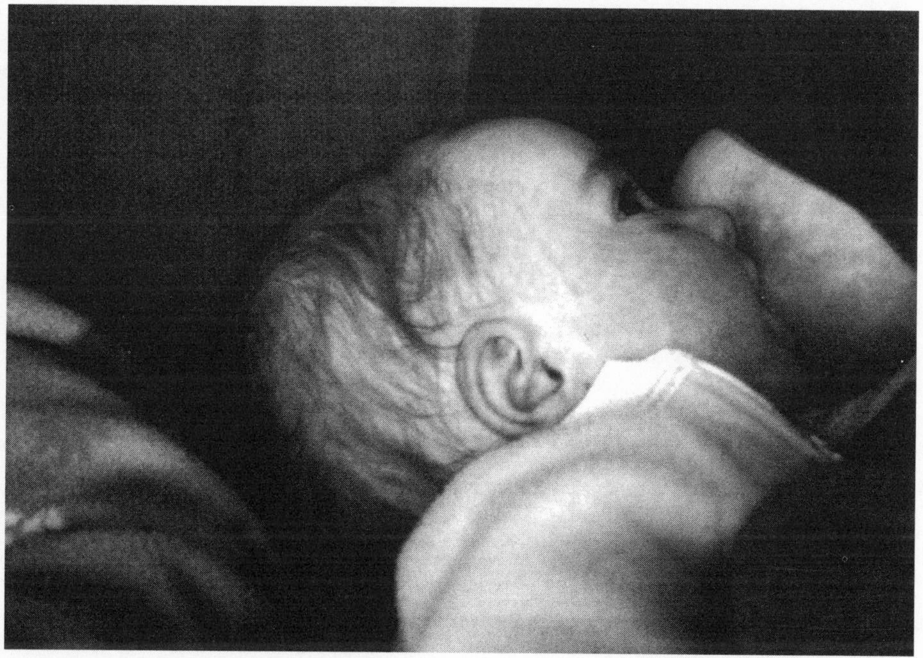

Breast tissue is soft and pliable, so it conforms to the unique shape of the baby's mouth. With every suck, the nipple is pushed by the tongue against the soft bones of the roof of the mouth, and if the nipple is firm it can gradually force the bone up into a high, narrow arch.

when he woke at night (to discourage waking at night to breastfeed), plus the raisins he liked to nibble during the day. We stopped both these practices, took more care with teeth cleaning, and continued breastfeeding. Because we got it early the decay did not need treatment, and it did not get any worse.

Mary, mother of Tom, who was breastfed for three years

ARTIFICIAL NIPPLES

While breastfeeding is always best, if a mother needs to use a bottle on a regular basis how does she select a suitable artificial nipple? Unfortunately, there is no easy answer. No artificial nipple has the dynamic qualities of the human breast or the capacity to adapt to the shape and size of the individual infant's mouth. Despite manufacturers' extravagant claims, no artificial nipple has been shown to be more like breastfeeding in every regard, or less likely to cause suck confusion in the newborn period, or to be potentially less damaging to the oral cavity. None have orthodontic benefits.

Most parents who use bottles say they try several types of nipples before they find one that suits their baby. Mothers should try to find a nipple that encourages the baby to open his mouth wide and is long enough to reach deep into his mouth. During breastfeeding a mother's nipple reaches the junction of the hard and soft palates at the back of the baby's mouth. This is approximately the length of two joints on an adult pinky. A softer, broader nipple is probably less likely to mold the roof of the mouth than a narrow, stiff nipple.

If breastfeeding is well established first, and the artificial nipple broad, soft, and deep in the mouth, the baby is more likely to transfer breastfeeding mouth actions and muscles when feeding from the bottle nipple. This is less likely to affect the mouth and will make it easier to switch back and forth from breast to bottle.

The mouths of babies are soft and malleable. They should be treated gently and with care. For the mouth, as in so many other ways, breast is best.

Ros Escott, I.B.C.L.C. is an occupational therapist, a lactation consultant, and a breastfeeding counselor with the Nursing Mothers' Association of Australia. She lives in Tasmania, Australia, and has one son. Her interest in the mouths of babies has been stimulated by the work of Chele Marmet, local speech pathologists, and three far-flung members of the dental profession, one in the United States, one in Brazil, and one in Ireland. Ros is particularly keen to see the WHO International Code of Marketing of Breast-milk Substitutes implemented in relation to feeding bottles and nipples, and the development of a worldwide standard to ensure quality and require information and warnings on labels. Hobbies? Ros collects strange and wonderful samples of bottles and nipples.

This detailed chapter on caring for breast milk is of special interest to women who must work outside their homes and need to know precisely how to care for their breast milk. Here are detailed instructions by a distinguished nutritionist.

Chapter 6
The Storage and Handling of Breast Milk

Robert G. Jensen, Ph.D.

Women who are nursing their infants often think they must stop because they must work outside their homes. However, they can feed the babies their own milk from a bottle by collecting and storing the milk. In this review, I will discuss accepted procedures for expression and storage of milk. My discussion is based upon a paper by Dr. Marget Hamosh, information from Ameda/Egnell, and a review by Lois D. W. Arnold. Working nursing mothers are also discussed in chapter 9 "What Every Breastfeeding Employee Should Know".

MICROORGANISMS

The major problem in the storage of milk is control of microorganisms. Microorganisms, including viruses, yeasts, protoza, and bacteria—or germs—are the microscopic cells that are found almost everywhere. Microorganisms that affect us grow best in conditions that humans find comfortable: 37° C, pH 6 to 8, water, an oxygen atmosphere, and suitable nutrients (substrates). Human and bovine (the class of animals that includes cows) milks are ideal substrates for the growth of harmless and pathogenic microorganisms. With optimal conditions, they can divide every twenty minutes (generation time), so that one cell becomes two, two four, and so on, until at the end of 4 hours, we can theoretically have 4,096 cells.

Bacteria in milk are often counted using the plate-count method. This procedure is an official method for analysis of bovine milk. The milk is diluted and mixed with a liquid substrate containing agar that is poured into flat, round, capped petri dishes. The agar solidifies, the plates are incubated at 37° C for up to twenty-four hours, and the colonies that have grown are counted. The results are now reported as colony-forming units (CFU) per millileter. There are many special substrates that will identify particular types of bacteria, such as *Eschericia coli (E. coli)* or *coliform*. Other methods are available that will provide total numbers of bacteria more rapidly. By determining the number of bacteria we can assess the sanitary status of milk and the procedures used to control bacterial growth, remove the bacteria, and reduce or destroy them.

Since large numbers of bacteria in milk indicate careless habits of procurement, we try to prevent their entry. Since bacterial growth is inhibited by low temperature, refrigeration is used to control it. Conversely, higher temperatures, as used in pasteurization (63.5° C for 30 minutes), will reduce the numbers of pathogens and destroy them. Milk can be sterilized at 121° C for 15 minutes to eliminate all bacteria, but since loss of important substances in milk occurs with heating (increasing with the length of time and temperature), these treatments are not used for the type of storage I am discussing.

Bacteria in human milk enter from the breast cells, skin, and nipples. They can be native or transferred by anything that touches the surfaces of clothes, wash cloths, sponges, dirty water, hands, faucet and refrigerator handles, cutting boards, and so on. Any of these surfaces that have residues of food will also have significant numbers of bacteria. If they have contacted fecal or decayed material, they can contain pathogens such as strains of *E. coli* that cause diarrhea. The only protection is to treat everything that will contact the milk or the baby as if it is contaminated.

Milk usually contains relatively small numbers of bacteria, less than 1000/ml, and these are mostly harmless skin types. I have listed the procedures for control of microorganisms in Table 6-1.

PREPARATION OF THE BREAST

The skin of the breast has microorganisms—normal inhabitants—that are harmless. However, bacteria that cause diseases can be carried to the breast by hands, clothing, and so on as discussed earlier unless care (good housekeeping) is employed.

For the greatest safety, then, breastfeeding mothers should be given the following instructions. The first step, and a must, is to wash the hands with a soap containing a bactericide. Pathogenic microorganisms, such as the recently identified lethal strain of *E. coli*, originate from fecal material. They can be transmitted from the bathroom to the breast and then to the infant by people who do not wash their hands after going to the toilet. Washing the hands should be a regular habit in all circumstances.

Then clean the breast with a mild soap that can contain a bactericide, but must be free of perfumes. One class of perfumes, the nitromusks, has been used in soaps and found in human milk. The breast is then disinfected with a mild bactericide, then rinsed and dried. The general purpose of the procedure is to remove bacteria from the skin by washing and destroying as many of them as possible with the bactericide.

MILK EXPRESSION

Milk is expressed from the breast by (a) manual massage, (b) a hand pump, or (c) an electric pump. A hand pump is the least desirable of the methods, because the rubber bulb on the bicycle horn type, is difficult to clean. If it is not clean it can be a significant source of bacteria. Manual expression does not remove as much milk as the electric pumps but bacterial contents can be kept low. The electric pumps must be cleaned. They remove more milk and fat than the other methods or than the baby does when nursing. Electric pumps are discussed by Walker and Auerbach and instructions for use by Ameda/Egnell. See also other chapters in this book.

Milk should be collected at the time the baby usually nurses to help stimulate and maintain the milk supply.

MILK COLLECTION

The entire contents of the breast can be collected or a few milliliters can be stripped and then the contents removed. The purpose of stripping and discarding about 5 milliliters is to remove excessive bacteria that may grow in the milk retained in the nipple between nursings. The current belief is that if nursing is regular, every three to four hours, stripping need not be done because the number of bacteria will not have had time to increase greatly. Discarding 5 milliliters of milk at each nursing could reduce the daily amount consumed by the infant by about 750 milliliters by 40 milliliters, or 5.3%. Even with infrequent nursing, stripping need not be done. I discussed procedures for washing the hands and breast above. These also apply to the pumps and storage containers.

STORAGE CONDITIONS

Containers

Milk can be stored in glass, hard plastic, or reinforced plastic containers. Glass containers are preferred. The lids for the glass container should have plastic liners. Both containers should have a permanent sticker or area that can be written

Table 6-1. Procedures in the Collection and Storage of Human Milk for Control of Microorganisms

1. Prevention of entry. Shielding important surfaces, nipple and surrounding skin; removal of bacteria from anything that will touch these surfaces.
2. Removal. Wash all skin surfaces with a mild soap, rinse, and disinfect; wash all metal, glass, and plastic surfaces that will touch milk with a detergent. Rinse, and disinfect. Washing will remove most microorganisms so a dishwasher can be used.
3. Destruction. Use of bactericides such as Phisohex.
4. Prevention of growth. Storage at low temperatures in the refrigerator or freezer.

on with a pencil. The marking material in pencils is graphite, not lead, so parents do not need to worry about lead getting into the milk. Ink or wax pencil marks may blur when the milk is stored in the refrigerator or freezer. Protective cells and other components in milk do not adhere to these container surfaces. The plastic bags are available from Medela/Avena.

Time and Temperature

Pasteurization of milk by heating in Pyrex glass bottles to, and holding at, 62.5° C (146° F) for 30 minutes destroys all pathogens, but also eliminates or reduces the amounts of useful components in milk, such as some immunoglobulins. Also pasteurization of a few bottles in the home is essentially impossible, since a container of milk must be totally immersed in a reliable water bath that will maintain the temperature at 62.5° C for 30 minutes. I have listed the types of storage that can be used in Table 6-2.

Mature milk can be left at room temperature for up to 8 hours, twelve to twelve hours for colostrum. Components in the milk inhibit bacterial growth. This procedure is convenient for the busy mother. However, if a large number of bacteria enter milk at some point, the number at the end of 8 hours would be high. We have seen that milk is an ideal medium for bacterial growth, so the generation time would be rapid, e.g., 20 minutes for one to become two, etc. Cleanliness is all important in preventing the entry of microorganisms into milk.

The refrigerator will maintain a temperature of 4° C (39.2° F). The growth of microorganisms is slower at this temperature and milk can be held for eight days. The bacterial count may increase somewhat, but this is not significant if the initial count is low. After storage the milk should be warmed to 38° C under warm water and shaken to redistribute the cream layer that forms when milk is left

Table 6-2. Times and Temperatures for Storage of Human Milk to Control Bacterial Growth.†

1. Room temperature. Up to 8 hours, useful if milk has not been contaminated. Convenient for the mother.
2. Refrigerator. 8 days at 4° C (39° F). Growth of bacteria is slowed at low temperatures.
3. Freezer. Compartment inside a refrigerator for 2 weeks. Refrigerated freezer with a separate door, -10° C (14° F) for 3 to 4 months. Deep freezer, -17° C (0° F) for 6 months or longer.

† *Milk to be used by healthy term infants.*

standing. The cream layer forms because the fat that is in small globules is lighter than water and will rise to the top. If the cream is not redistributed, a large difference in the fat content of the milk layers will occur, high at the top, low at the bottom. The original bacterial count may be decreased in some samples. Milk contains a variety of components and mechanisms that can inhibit or destroy microorganisms. One of these is a lipase, or fat-splitting, enzyme that, if activated, will produce microbicidal compounds.

Milk can be stored for two weeks in a freezer compartment located inside a refrigerator, three to four months in a refrigerator/freezer with a separate door at -10° C (14° F), or 6 months or longer in a deep freezer at −17° C (0° F) . Bacterial growth is virtually nil at these temperatures, but milk lipase is still active, although the reaction time is reduced. If the lipase has been activated, compounds will be released that may produce a tallowy off-flavor. If this is tasted by the infant, the milk may be rejected.

Table 6-3. Steps Needed for Collection, Storage, and Use of Human Milk.†

1. Clean and disinfect hands, breast, etc., and pump parts that will touch the breast.
2. Pump or hand express milk at the same time nursing would have occurred to maintain lactation schedule.
3. Store labeled glass bottle or approved plastic bag as follows:
   a. Room temperature, up to 8 hours.
   b. Refrigerator, up to 8 days.
   c. Freezer, 2 weeks to 6 months, depending on type of freezer.
4. Warm milk to 38° C (97° F), mix thoroughly, smell and taste, and mix thoroughly. Do not use microwave to thaw frozen milk. Use the oldest milk first.

† *Milk to be used by healthy term infants.*

My discussion has probably made the storage of milk more complicated than it is in practice. The steps required for proper storage are listed in Table 6-3. If this protocol is followed, the milk should be safe for consumption by the infant. The almost routine separation of mother and child has resulted in a culture where there are many women who pump or express their milk for future use. Knowing the procedures for storage and handling ensures that milk given to the infant is healthy. Once a mother understands the issues and develops a routine, providing breast milk to her child when she is away is safe and easy.

Robert G. Jensen, Ph.D., is the editor and a contributor to the *Handbook of Milk Composition,* published by Academic Press in 1995, and is noted for his research on fats in bovine and human milks. He earned his B.S., M.S., and Ph.D. degrees from the University of Missouri. He is a professor emeritus at the University of Connecticut, Department of Animal Industries. Dr. Jensen is married and has two adult sons.

Section Two

Matters for Moms

Becoming a parent brings changes to many areas of people's lives, and one of the major areas is often that of sex. For professionals working with parents who find no problems in resuming their sex lives after the birth of a baby this chapter may not be needed, but for those who help people who thought they were alone it can bring a breath of fresh air.

Chapter 7
Sex and the Breastfeeding Woman

Wendy Brodribb, A.M., M.B.B.S., I.B.C.L.C.

There are always changes when people become parents. Not only is there a new dependent person to care for, but the relationships between the mother and father, with other family members, and with friends will change. At times, these changes create unanticipated difficulties in these relationships, particularly with the mother's partner. Even before a pregnancy, sex is sometimes a difficult subject, and this is often accentuated by the birth of a child.

Unfortunately the changes that having a baby can bring to a couple's sex life are rarely discussed, and yet many couples have concerns about what is normal and what effects they can anticipate. Healthcare professionals should bring up these issues with new parents.

Most parents have fears and questions about making love after the birth. When is it okay to start having sex again? Traditionally women have been told to wait for six weeks after the birth, but this depends on the particular woman and any difficulties with the birth. Will it hurt? Will it be the same as before? Will the mother's response be the same?

Parents should be aware that:

- There is nearly always a change in a sexual relationship following the birth of a baby.
- Many couples find they don't enjoy intercourse for a least two months after birth, and for some couples it is even longer.
- Even after a year many couples have intercourse less often than before the pregnancy, even if the baby has been weaned.
- Women often find their interest in sex is less than their partner's.

- Some women find that their libido only returns with the onset of regular menstruation following their baby's birth, which usually means after weaning.
- In the long term, however, many women report their interest in sex is higher after adjustments to the baby are made than it was before their pregnancy.

FATIGUE

Almost everyone feels tired in the days and weeks following the birth of a baby. The pregnancy and birth are hard work, as is caring for a newborn. With disturbed nights and a reduced amount of sleep for both parents, sex is often the last thing either parent wants to think about at the end of the day. Tiredness is the most common reason given by parents for reduced sexual desire and response.

PAIN

Many women experience pain or discomfort making love the first time after the birth. This is more likely if there has been an episiotomy or stitches. These take time to heal and scarring takes time to soften and stretch. Hemorrhoids, anal fissures, and vaginal varices (dilated blood vessels in the vaginal wall) may also hurt.

Up to fifty percent of women report they are still experiencing some discomfort with intercourse up to five months following the birth of their baby. However, continuing pain is not normal. This needs to be checked by an expert.

Because of the hormones released during breastfeeding, estrogen levels may be low, and this in turn may cause the vagina to be dry and the amount of lubrication during sex to be reduced. Sometimes this leads to pain during intercourse, especially during penetration.

CHANGE IN BODY SHAPE

Changes to a woman's body following her pregnancy may affect the way she and her partner feel about sex. A woman may find that her hips and thighs are broader than before. Fat laid down during pregnancy stores energy for breastfeeding and is gradually used up in the first few months of the baby's life.

Breasts also change in shape and size and may feel full and tender, especially in the first few weeks. Sometimes milk leaks from the breasts, especially during orgasm. Some couples find breast changes during lactation particularly erotic, while others find them offensive. Couples should be reassured that there is no "right" or "wrong."

Both stomach muscles and those around the vagina (pelvic floor) have usually been stretched, and take a while to get back the tone they had previously. Exercises to strengthen abdominal and pelvic floor muscles are often taught postnatally, and are well worth doing regularly. Strong pelvic floor muscles help both partners enjoy sex more.

HORMONAL CHANGES

During pregnancy levels of estrogen and progesterone as well as many other hormones are very high. After the baby is born, the levels of these hormones fall quite dramatically, and then return to the pre-pregnant state by about three months in women who are not breastfeeding. However, in women who are breastfeeding, estrogen and progesterone levels may not reach their pre-pregnant levels for many months. This is usually linked with delayed ovulation and the first menstrual period.

Low estrogen levels may also reduce sexual desire. Sexual arousal may occur more slowly and be less intense, lubrication is slower and less profuse, the vaginal walls are thinner, distension slower and less marked.

On the other hand, for some women the libido increases during breastfeeding. Breastfeeding can be a sexually pleasurable experience, since oxytocin—a hormone released at the time of milk ejection—is also released during orgasm. Either response is within the normal range.

PSYCHOLOGICAL FACTORS

Many women feel a sense of wholeness and womanliness enhancing their sexual attractiveness and well-being after the birth of their baby. This often brings a time of peace and maturing while other women feel some conflict over the roles of mother, lover, and partner, sometimes leading to an emotional roller-coaster ride that may reduce libido. These women may experience emotions such as fear, anxiety, low self-esteem, depression, guilt or resentment. In some cases, professional intervention may be needed.

Sometimes the close skin-to-skin contact a mother has with her baby when she's feeding, cuddling, soothing, and nurturing him or her provides the mother with all the closeness that she needs—she might feel "touched out." Occasionally, this is at an emotional rather than at a physical level. By giving so much to others (children and partner), she may have nothing to give in a sexual way, wanting time and space for herself. Both mother and partner may be so totally immersed and in love with the baby that sex is a very unimportant area of their lives. The partner's feeling may change too. He may feel very protective of the mother and baby and avoid sex for that reason.

Postnatal depression almost always causes a loss of sexual desire and response as well as a lack of enjoyment in life in general. Depression of this type may require professional help. Once the depression improves, mothers find that they also become more interested in sex again.

RELATIONSHIP FACTORS

After the birth of a baby mother and partner are never the same again. Their feelings, fears, desires, and needs change, often in a positive way; nevertheless these changes can cause conflict within a relationship if not openly discussed.

WILL WEANING HELP?

Many of the changes to the mother's body and in how she feels about herself will occur whether she is breastfeeding or not, so weaning the baby early is not a magic way to return to her pre-pregnant self. Breastfeeding also has many positive benefits for her, her baby, and her family. Whether or not she continues to breastfeed if there are sexual problems, there must be a balance between these factors.

During the time when the baby is young, intercourse may not be as important as it was previously, but to be held, cuddled, kissed, and nurtured is often more important than before. Couples should be able to express their love and caring for each other without the pressure to perform and have intercourse. Doing so often lets them relax and feel more positive about their sexuality.

PLAN AHEAD

Babies have the uncanny knack of waking up just when their parents are about to have sex, so spontaneity is often a thing of the past—for a while anyway. Having sex soon after the baby has been fed usually means that the baby falls and stays asleep, and the mother's breasts are less full and uncomfortable. Some couples wait until after the early-morning feed, when they have had a bit more sleep too.

Sometimes it is difficult for a mother to turn off the mother side of herself and become the lover. Coming to bed relaxed, and feeling good about herself—how she looks and who she is—may help. Attractive nightwear, perfume, and soft lights can add an aura of romance. If the initial contact is not sexual—perhaps a massage—it will be less threatening, and more relaxing. Neither partner should worry about performance. The aim is for both to enjoy the sexual encounter. Whether this involves intercourse or orgasm is not important.

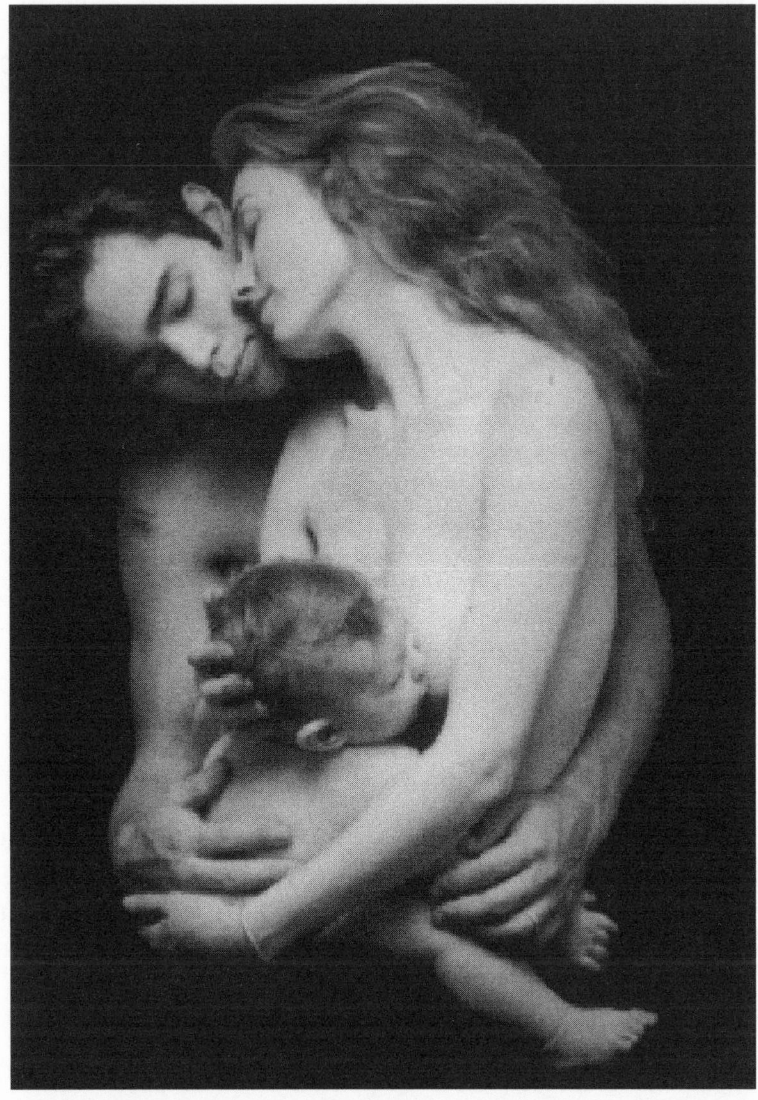

Having a baby almost always brings changes in a couple's sexual relationship. However, the adjustment period can be eased by communication and loving understanding on the part of both partners. Photograph by Michele-Salimeri, New York,, NY.

MINIMIZING PAIN AND DISCOMFORT

The vagina is designed to become lubricated as part of the sexual buildup before intercourse. This aids the penetration of the penis, and reduces discomfort. Vaginal lubrication may be affected by how the mother feels (again switching her mind onto sex will help) and by the hormonal changes in her body. Many breast-feeding women have lower estrogen levels than before they were pregnant, and this tends to make the vaginal walls a little thinner and lubrication a little slower. It may help to wait longer before penetration than previously or to use a vaginal lubricant.

Vaginal tears or episiotomy scars take a while to heal, and may also cause pain or discomfort, especially during the first few sexual encounters. Stretching the vagina by gently massaging with two fingers around the base of the vaginal opening, and consciously relaxing the vagina before having sex, may help. Some positions cause less pressure on the scar.

Cesarean section or tubal ligation scars can also hurt and a new position may prove more comfortable.

Breasts and nipples tend to be more sensitive than before, especially during the early weeks of breastfeeding. This may cause difficulties if the woman's breasts have played a big role in her sex life before the baby was born. She should be encouraged to talk to her partner about what feels comfortable for her now. As the baby gets older, she will probably find that her breasts no longer feel uncomfortable or leak milk as frequently.

TIMING

There is no competition about when couples start having sex again, although the doctor should make a suggestion. Some couples are eager to resume intercourse as soon as possible, others feel happier waiting for weeks or months. When the time does come, couples should give themselves plenty of time to experiment, and take things slowly. This tends to make the whole experience more pleasurable and less stressful for both. This may be the time to find new ways of pleasuring each other and new ways of communicating.

WHAT NEXT?

When a couple has a new baby, sex may not have top priority. But this period does not last, and they can look forward to a time when sex will be just as good as before they had the baby, if not better. Meanwhile, both enjoy the different rewards that come with this stage of life.

Wendy Brodribb, A.M., M.B.B.S., I.B.C.L.C., has been a doctor in Queensland, Australia, for over twenty years. She became a counselor for the Nursing Mother's Association of Australia (N.M.A.A.) in 1983, and a lactation consultant (I.B.C.L.C.) in 1990. She has been actively involved in N.M.A.A., serving on the board of directors for five years, and was its national president in 1994 and 1995. She has published a number of papers on breastfeeding and is editor for both editions of *Breastfeeding Management* in Australia.

Very few people are unaware of the benefits of breastfeeding to the baby, but the many benefits to the mother are often overlooked or even not known. From the effect of oxytocin on the uterus to the warm emotional gains, breastfeeding gives the mother many reasons to be pleased with her choice. These are outlined here in a professional presentation.

Chapter 8

A Well-Kept Secret: Breastfeeding's Benefits to Mothers

Alicia Dermer, M.D., I.B.C.L.C.

One of the best-kept secrets about breastfeeding is that it's as healthy for mothers as for babies. Not only does lactation continue the natural physiologic process begun with conception and pregnancy, but it provides many short- and long-term health benefits. These issues are rarely emphasized in prenatal counseling by healthcare professionals and all but ignored in popular parenting literature. Let's look at all the benefits breastfeeding provides mothers and speculate as to why so few are finding out about it.

PHYSIOLOGIC EFFECTS OF BREASTFEEDING

Immediately after birth, the repeated suckling of the baby releases oxytocin from the mother's pituitary gland. This hormone not only signals the breasts to release milk to the baby (this is known as the milk-ejection reflex, or "letdown"), but simultaneously produces contractions in the uterus. The resulting contractions prevent postpartum hemorrhage and promote uterine involution.

Bottle-feeding mothers frequently get synthetic oxytocin at birth through an intravenous line, but for the next few days, during which they are at highest risk of postpartum hemorrhage, they are on their own.

As long as a mother breastfeeds without substituting formula, foods, or pacifiers for feedings at the breast, the return of her menstrual periods is delayed. Unlike bottle-feeding mothers, who typically get their periods back within six to eight weeks, breastfeeding mothers can often stay amenorrheic for several months. This condition has the important benefits of preserving iron in the mother's body and often provides natural spacing of pregnancies.

The amount of iron a mother's body uses in milk production is much less than the amount she would lose from menstrual bleeding. The net effect is a decreased risk of iron-deficiency anemia in the breastfeeding mother as compared with her formula-feeding counterpart. The longer the mother nurses and keeps her periods at bay, the stronger this effect.

As for fertility, the lactational amenorrhea method (LAM) is a well-documented contraceptive method, with ninety-eight to ninety-nine percent prevention of pregnancy in the first six months. The bottle-feeding mother needs to start contraception within six weeks of the birth. The natural child-spacing achieved through LAM ensures the optimal survival of each child and the physical recovery of the mother between pregnancies.

If LAM cannot be used to its fullest extent or if the mother wishes additional protection, most contraceptive methods, including barrier methods, IUDs and progesterone-only hormonal contraceptives, are compatible with breastfeeding.

LONG-TERM BENEFITS OF BREASTFEEDING

It is now becoming clear that breastfeeding provides mothers with more than just short-term benefits in the early period after birth. A number of studies have shown other potential health advantages that mothers can enjoy through breastfeeding. These include optimal metabolic profiles, reduced risk of various cancers, and psychological benefits.

Production of milk is an active metabolic process, requiring the use of calories—two hundred to five hundred per day, on average. To use up this many calories, a bottle-feeding mother would have to swim at least thirty laps in a pool or bicycle uphill for an hour daily. Clearly, breastfeeding mothers have an edge on losing that pregnancy weight gain, and studies have confirmed that formula-feeding mothers lose less weight and don't keep it off as well as breastfeeding mothers.

The above finding is particularly important for mothers who have had diabetes during their pregnancies. After birth, mothers with a history of gestational diabetes who breastfeed have lower blood sugars than nonbreastfeeding mothers. For these women, who are already at increased risk of developing diabetes, the optimal weight loss from breastfeeding may translate into a decreased risk of diabetes in later life.

Women with Type I diabetes prior to their pregnancies tend to need less insulin while they breastfeed due to their reduced sugar levels. Breastfeeding mothers tend to have a high HDL cholesterol. The optimal weight loss, improved blood sugar control, and good cholesterol profile provided by breastfeeding may ultimately pay off with a lower risk of heart problems. This is especially important since heart attacks are the leading cause of death in women.

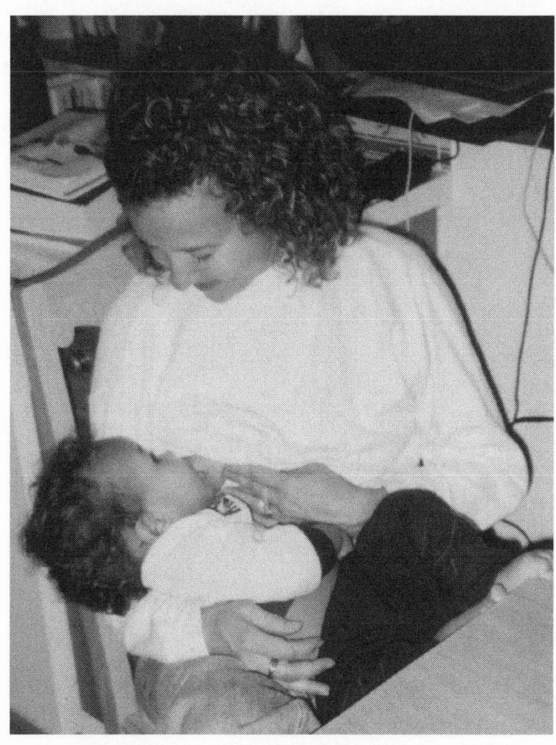

Breastfeeding provides a special interaction between a child and her mother. Bottle-feeding mothers must work hard to replicate it. As the child breast-feeds, its mother's breast produces a special hormonal milieu. What's more, prolactin, the milk-making hormone, appears to produce a special calmness in the mother.

Another important element used in producing milk is calcium. Because women lose calcium while lactating, some health professionals have mistakenly assigned an increased risk of osteoporosis to breastfeeding. However, current studies show that after weaning their children, breastfeeding mothers have a return of their bone density to normal or even higher levels. In the long term, lactation may actually result in stronger bones and reduced risk of osteoporosis. In fact, recent studies have confirmed that women who did not breastfeed have a higher risk of hip fractures after menopause.

Nonbreastfeeding mothers have been shown in numerous studies to have a higher risk of reproductive cancers. Ovarian and uterine cancers have been found to be more common in women who did not breastfeed. This may be due to the repeated ovulatory cycles and exposure to higher levels of estrogen from not breastfeeding. Although numerous studies have looked at the relationship between breastfeeding and breast cancer, the results have been conflicting. This is largely due to flaws in study design and lack of uniform definition of breastfeeding, resulting in difficulty comparing the data. Despite this, it is now estimated that breastfeeding from six to twenty-four months throughout a mother's reproductive lifetime may reduce the risk of breast cancer by eleven to twenty-five percent. This phenomenon may also be due to suppressed ovulation and low estrogen, but a local effect relating to the normal physiologic function of the breast may also be involved. This was suggested by a study in which mothers who traditionally breastfed on only one side had significantly higher rates of cancer in the unsuckled breast.

DOES BREASTFEEDING PHYSICALLY HARM MOTHERS?

In two studies, there appeared to be an increase in flare-ups of rheumatoid arthritis in breastfeeding mothers. However, in another study, overall severity and mortality of rheumatoid arthritis was worse in women who had never breastfed. So even with this condition, it's not clear whether breastfeeding harms. There have been no other studies showing any detrimental health effects to women from breastfeeding. Bottom line: Breastfeeding reduces the risk of three of the biggest killers of women—female cancers, heart disease, and osteoporosis—without any significant health risks.

PSYCHOLOGICAL ISSUES FOR BREASTFEEDING MOTHERS

How do you measure the peace of mind of having a healthy baby who is developing optimally? How do you quantify the increased stress on formula-feeding mothers of recurrent ear infections, increased costs of feeding the baby, development of chronic illnesses such as asthma, diabetes, or cancer, which are more likely in formula-fed babies? Where do you factor in the financial burden of formula prices and increased medical costs?

Public health agencies advocate for breastfeeding because of its well-documented health advantages to babies, but they fail to convey to individual mothers and families the potential emotional impact of this very crucial infant-feeding decision. In our society, the decision about breast or bottle is still seen very much as a personal choice based on convenience. The potential stress of living with a child with recurrent illnesses, or the loss of the unique bond that comes from breastfeeding, are often omitted from the decision-making process.

There is much more to breastfeeding than the provision of optimal nutrition and protection from disease through mother's milk. Breastfeeding provides a unique interaction between mother and child, an automatic, skin-to-skin closeness and nurturing that bottle-feeding mothers have to work to replicate. The child's suckling at the breast produces a special hormonal milieu for the mother. Prolactin, the milk-making hormone, appears to produce a special calmness in mothers. Breastfeeding mothers have been shown to have a less intense response to adrenaline.

This calming effect is hard to measure in a society largely unsupportive of breastfeeding such as the United States, where breastfeeding beyond a few weeks is not the norm. Mothers who try to breastfeed in this climate often experience physical and emotional problems. Physical problems result from a lack of breastfeeding role models among family and friends, compounded by the easy availability of formula and a lack of access to knowledgeable supportive healthcare professionals.

Even if a mother overcomes physical problems, she may still encounter negative comments, such as "Are you still nursing?" or "Your milk may not be strong enough—why don't you add formula?" Or her boss may make it impossible for her to continue breastfeeding on returning to work. Or she may be harassed for breastfeeding in public. No wonder that few mothers get to fully experience the relaxing effects of breastfeeding.

New motherhood is a time fraught with emotion. Postpartum depression is common, often exacerbated by lack of support and a sense of isolation. The role of breastfeeding in postpartum emotional upheavals has not been well studied, but breastfeeding mothers with depression need treatment just as much as any other mother.

They present a unique challenge to healthcare professionals. Since most medications pass into breast milk, many physicians believe the safest solution is to wean the child. However, in most cases of depression, women do better if they continue to breastfeed. Unfortunately, too often physicians insist that mothers wean their child in order to take antidepressant medicines.

A review of the literature, however, has demonstrated that several antidepressants pose minimal, if any, risk to the nursing child. A mother who feels that her nursing relationship with her child is the only thing going right in her life can now continue to breastfeed while receiving appropriate medications for her depression.

WHY DON'T MORE PEOPLE KNOW HOW GOOD BREASTFEEDING IS?

Clearly, breastfeeding is good for mothers both physically and emotionally. And yet, many mothers decide to breastfeed based solely on the benefits to the baby. Breastfeeding in the context of a bottle-feeding society tends to be perceived as inconvenient and uncomfortable.

Often, mothers see breastfeeding as a martyrdom to be endured for their baby's health. If they stop early, they may feel guilty about depriving the baby of some health benefits, but their guilt is often soothed by well-meaning people who reassure them that "baby will do just as well on formula." Perhaps if they knew that continuing to breastfeed is also good for their own health, some mothers might be less likely to quit when they run into problems.

Many mothers are not being told how good breastfeeding is for their health. Whether out of ignorance or due to the influence of the artificial baby milk industry, healthcare professionals fail to inform mothers of the facts. It's time for this well-kept secret to come out. Hopefully, as word spreads about these little-known facts, more mothers will not merely choose to breastfeed briefly to provide early disease protection for their baby, but will continue to breastfeed, providing optimal outcomes both for their children and for themselves.

RESOURCES FOR NEW PARENTS

Depression After Delivery (DAD)
1-800-944-4773
Staffed by volunteer healthcare professionals and support groups nationwide

Postpartum Education for Parents (PEP)
1-805-564-3888
Twenty-four-hour "warm line" that new parents can call with questions about the postpartum period and newborn care

La Leche League International
1-800-525-3243
Twenty-four-hour line providing mother-to-mother breastfeeding support

---

Alicia Dermer, M.D., I.B.C.L.C., is Clinical Associate Professor in the Department of Family Medicine at the University of Medicine and Dentistry of New Jersey–Robert Wood Johnson Medical School in New Brunswick, New Jersey. She has a special interest in wellness and health promotion. As part of this interest, she has gained expertise in breastfeeding education and promotion. She successfully sat for the certifying examination of the International Board of Lactation Examiners in 1995. She lectures extensively on the subject of lactation, is actively involved in healthcare professional and lay education about breastfeeding, and has several publications in the medical literature on the subject.

Section Three

Breastfeeding in the Real World

Very few new mothers today have the luxury of staying home with their babies. Instead, when their maternity leave, however long or short it may be, is over, they must return to work. This chapter discusses both the role of the law and of society in helping the breastfeeding mother return to work while continuing to breastfeed.

Chapter 9
What Every Breastfeeding Employee Should Know

Naomi Bromberg Bar-Yam, Ph.D.

In the spring of 1998, a court in Oregon awarded a woman $280,000 in lost wages and damages against her former employer. The reason? The company denied her time to breastfeed her baby on the job. While this represents a dawning awareness of the importance of breastfeeding, there is still much more legal work to be done.

Today, the fact that two of three mothers are employed by others has inspired changes in the laws that support a worker's family obligations, whether it is leave for new fathers, on-site childcare, or accommodations for breastfeeding for a new mother.

Over half the women who are employed when they become pregnant return to the labor force by the time their children are three months old, in keeping with general maternity leave policies. This has inspired new laws supporting a worker's family obligations, including leave for new fathers and, of special interest to readers of this book, accommodations for breastfeeding for mothers.

BREASTFEEDING LEGISLATION

In Florida, Minnesota, and Texas, the rights of new mothers to breastfeed at work have been recognized through statewide legislation. Other states and the federal government are considering legislation that would mandate that employees provide arrangements for women to work and nurse their children. Until the time when all employees encourage breastfeeding, however, the breastfeeding worker can use a variety of techniques to care for her child and accomplish her work-related tasks.

Many businesses today accommodate employees who are continuing to breastfeed their babies at home. Special "Nursing Mothers' Rooms" provide comfort as well as privacy for those women who wish to use a breast pump in order to get breast milk that they will carry home at the end of the day. Photograph reproduced by permission of Medela, Inc.

WHAT IS COMPANY POLICY?

Increasing competition has made it beneficial for companies to offer generous benefits in order to retain their best workers. One of those benefits is flexibility in the work schedule. Women presently working a straight eight-hour day may be able to change their schedule. Flextime, part-time, and job-sharing plans were not invented to accommodate nursing mothers, but they are good for the breastfeeding employee, nonetheless.

Human resources, benefits, and work-and-life departments in large companies can guide a new mother through the workplace possibilities for nursing while working. Maternity leave can be as long as three months or six months. The mother has to consider plans for professional advancement and the family's need for money as well as how much time she wants to spend with her new baby.

More and more women want to juggle working, parenting, and breastfeeding. They should be advised to talk about it with their co-workers, family members, and company supervisors early. Unfortunately, many companies offer generous work/family benefits while at the same time creating a workplace culture that makes it very difficult for women (and men) to use them.

Today's working mothers are committed to being both good workers and good mothers, but they can only accomplish this when they have the support that they need in the workplace and at home. Company policies are beginning to reflect this. Flexibility and open communication are key. It is important for mothers and supervisors to engage in an ongoing conversation throughout the transition back to work to ensure they are working together.

NURSING AT WORK

Nursing mothers who are separated from their babies for long periods of time must find some other way to feed them during their absence. Most nursing working mothers in the United States use a breast pump to express breast milk while at work. This milk is stored to be fed their babies the next day in day care or at home by a caretaker. Four things are essential to establish successful workplace lactation: space, time, support, and gatekeepers.

• Space

Breastfeeding at work requires quiet, private space. Women who have their own private offices usually use them to express milk for their babies. However, women who do not have their own offices also have babies and continue to nurse them upon their return to work. Some companies have Nursing Mothers' Rooms (NMR), centrally located with privacy and, perhaps, a breast pump. Where there is no designated NMR, women often use spare conference rooms, offices, or even large closets.

Bathrooms are not acceptable places to pump! Women are not asked to eat lunch or drink coffee in a bathroom. It is unsanitary and inappropriate to pump milk or breastfeed in a bathroom.

If the baby is in on-site or near-site daycare, the mother can probably nurse the baby directly at least once a day, although it is usually necessary to pump as well.

• Time

Breastfeeding and breast-milk expression take time. The fully breastfeeding mother of an infant under four months will probably need to take three twenty-minute nursing breaks in an eight-hour work day. As the baby begins to take solid foods, between four and six months of age, breastfeeding will diminish. Even if they continue to nurse their babies, by nine to twelve months most mothers will no longer need to pump at work.

Many mothers choose to nurse or pump instead of eating lunch. This is bad for both mother and baby. It takes a lot of calories to nurse a baby. Unfortunately, taking time to pump at work may annoy co-workers and supervisors.

It should be stressed that nursing employees do not usually pump for more than a year and the time spent pumping is made up for by reduced absenteeism. In enlightened companies, corporate policies reflect that there is greater productivity and concentration on the job when a worker knows her baby is receiving the best

Table 9-1: Descriptions of Flexible Work Programs and Their Benefits for New Mothers and Employers:

EARNED TIME

Sick leave, vacation time and personal days are grouped into one set of paid days off. Workers take these days at their own discretion. Mothers do not have to justify time off to their supervisors. Often, earned time accrues over several years, giving new mothers substantial paid leave after birth. Promotes loyalty because workers feel trusted and valued. Workers often are willing to work extra time when necessary because company accommodates their needs.

PART-TIME

Workers work less than 35-40 hours/week. Benefits are usually prorated to hours worked. Gives new mothers more time at home. Often includes flexibility of which hours are worked. Retain workers with valuable experience and training. Saves recruiting and training new employees.

JOB SHARING

Two employees each work part-time and share the responsibilities and benefits of one job position. Gives mothers more time at home keeping the same job. Retain workers with experience. Keeps full time coverage of job.

PHASE BACK

Workers return from leave to full time work load gradually over several weeks or months. Longer return to work adjustment period for mother and baby. More time with infant, when breastfeeding is being established. Retains workers with experience. Promotes loyalty and dedication of workers. Keeps worker involved with job responsibilities.

FLEX-TIME

Workers arrange to work hours to suit their schedules, (i.e. seven am to three pm, or ten am –six pm.) Can work with spouse's schedule to require less paid child care. Can arrange hours around best times of day to be with baby. Shorter commutes in less traffic. Workplace covered for more hours per day. Workers are better able to focus when schedules better suit their needs. Less likely to need to leave early on a regular basis.

COMPRESSED WORK WEEK

Workers work more hours on fewer days, (i.e. seven am to seven pm for 3 days per week.) Allows new mothers full days at home with their babies. Workers better able to focus when schedules better suit their needs. Retains workers with experience and training. Employee still works full time hours.

TELECOMMUTING

Workers work all or part of their jobs from home. Can work around baby's schedule. Less commuting time. Less work clothing and travel expenses. Retains workers with experience and training. Saves office and parking space.

ON-SITE OR NEAR-SITE DAY CARE

Day care provided on or near site, often sponsored by the company. Can visit baby for nursing, etc., during the work day. Commuting time is with baby. Promotes loyalty among workers. Workers better able to focus when baby is accessible.

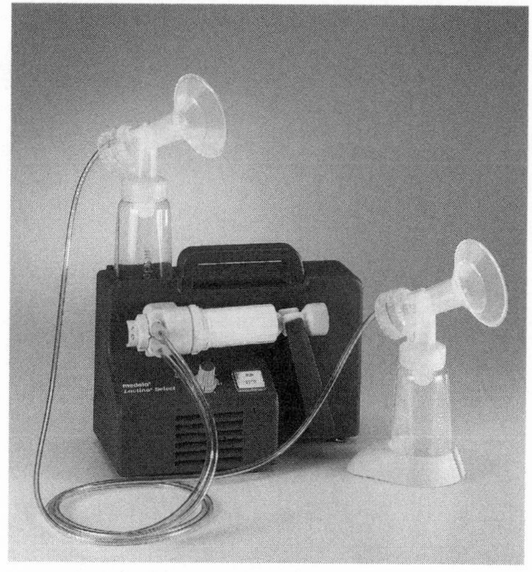

A breastpump with a sucking cycle of at least sixty times per minute, like this one by Medela, mimics the sucking of a baby. A high quality pump will keep the milk supply strong and will obtain the most milk in the least amount of time. Photograph reproduced by permission of Medela, Inc.

food possible. The discomfort of full breasts is relieved by pumping regularly, another practical reason for three twenty-minute breaks in each eight-hour shift.

• Support

All breastfeeding mothers, not just those employed outside the home, need support from as many places as possible. This can come from husbands, parents and in-laws, friends, healthcare providers and, of course, the workplace. Companies with the resources to implement lactation programs have discovered that accommodating nursing workers is good for the bottom line.

Over seventy-five companies, including Eastman Kodak, Cigna, Blue Cross–Blue Shield, CNN, and Home Depot, are trying, and liking, the results. One company estimates the company saves several thousand dollars and three days of sick leave annually for each breastfed baby in their program.

Workplaces that value women's roles in mothering as well as in employment increase workers' morale, productivity, loyalty, and dedication. Company-sponsored lactation programs are an excellent form of support for nursing mothers. In addition, new mothers often meet one another in the Nursing Mothers' Room or washing out pumps, providing informal support and sometimes forming the basis for support groups.

On the other hand, women who have no workplace lactation support have the opportunity to educate supervisors and co-workers about the benefits and feasibility of breastfeeding at work.

• Gatekeepers

Gatekeepers are those people in each workplace who make sure that time, space, and support all come together for the nursing mother. Sometimes, the most important gatekeeper is the human resources department that sets up the lactation support program.

In some companies, the supervisor makes sure that things in the department are flexible enough that new mothers can take the time and find the space they need to pump. In other places, the most important gatekeeper is the office manager or secretary, who knows which offices and conference rooms are empty and can arrange schedules so that the new mother can pump at ten and again at two or on her own schedule. Co-workers who cover for the nursing mother are invaluable gatekeepers, too.

VARIATIONS IN WORKPLACE LACTATION SUPPORT

There are many ways in which businesses support nursing employees. In some companies, it is the new mothers themselves who make their employers aware of their needs with the employers doing their best to accommodate them. Often they make some space, such as a spare office or conference room, available to these women. Usually, such arrangements are made within the department and do not involve company policy.

Good programs are represented by company-wide policies that support continued breastfeeding in the workplace. They have Nursing Mothers' Rooms (NMR) that have good lighting and ventilation, privacy (locking door or "occupied" sign), sink, electrical outlet, and often a refrigerator. Sometimes the company provides a hospital-grade breast pump and gives or sells personal supplies to the mother. Time, usually unpaid, is made available for mothers to express milk during the work day.

Some companies have a more elaborate lactation program with designated, equipped NMRs and unpaid time to pump or nurse. In addition, such programs include the services of a lactation consultant who meets with the mother as needed, beginning during her maternity leave, to help plan the transition back to the workplace, and continuing after her return to work to ease the adjustment to the new schedule and demands. The lactation consultant may be employed by the company or paid as an independent consultant. Sometimes the lactation consultant also provides education to expectant and new fathers. Some workplaces with lactation programs also have on-site or near-site daycare where mothers can nurse their babies during the day.

Table 9-2: Descriptions of Flexible Work Programs and Their Benefits for New Mothers and Employers

Earned time

Sick leave, vacation time and personal days are grouped into one set of paid days off. Workers take these days at their own discretion. Mothers do not have to justify time off to their supervisors. Often, earned time accrues over several years, giving new mothers substantial paid leave after birth. Promotes loyalty because workers feel trusted and valued. Workers often are willing to work extra time when necessary because company accommodates their needs.

Part-time

Workers work less than 35–40 hours/week. Benefits are usually prorated to hours worked. Gives new mothers more time at home. Often includes flexibility of which hours are worked. Retains workers with valuable experience and training. Saves recruiting and training new employees.

Job sharing

Two employees each work part-time and share the responsibilities and benefits of one job position. Gives mothers more time at home while keeping the same job. Retains workers with experience. Keeps full-time coverage of job.

Phase back

Workers return from leave to full-time work load gradually over several weeks or months. Longer return-to-work adjustment period for mother and baby. More time with infant, when breastfeeding is being established. Retains workers with experience. Promotes loyalty and dedication of workers. Keeps worker involved with job responsibilities.

Flex-time

Workers arrange to work hours to suit their schedules (i.e. seven a.m. to three p.m. or ten a.m. to six p.m.). Can work with spouse's schedule to require less paid childcare. Can arrange hours around best times of day to be with baby. Shorter commutes in less traffic. Workplace covered for more hours per day. Workers are better able to focus when schedules better suit their needs. Less likely to need to leave early on a regular basis.

Compressed work week

Workers work more hours on fewer days (i.e. seven a.m. to seven p.m. for 3 days per week). Allows new mothers full days at home with their babies. Workers better able to focus when schedules better suit their needs. Retains workers with experience and training. Employee still works full-time hours.

Telecommuting

Workers work all or part of their jobs from home. Can work around baby's schedule. Less commuting time. Less work clothing and travel expenses. Retains workers with experience and training. Saves office and parking space.

On-site or near-site day care

Day care provided on or near site, often sponsored by the company. Can visit baby for nursing, etc., during the work day. Commuting time is with baby. Promotes loyalty among workers. Workers better able to focus when baby is accessible.

Table 9-3. Worksheet for Discussing Return-to-Work Plan with Supervisor

This worksheet is a guide for a woman's ongoing conversation with her supervisor about nursing at work. All of the questions and concerns may not be relevant to each situation and there may be other concerns and questions that are. The employee should not worry if all the questions can't be answered in the first meeting. This is an ongoing conversation. Flexibility and open communication are the keys to success!

Plan:

What return-to-work plans are the mother and her supervisor considering? The questions below can be discussed about each plan or about all the plans being considered together.

Measuring success: By what criteria will she and her supervisor measure whether the plan is working? When and how will they discuss its success so that they can work out modifications and adjustments along the way?

Time and space: How will adjustments be made in the time worked to take into account her needs as a nursing mother? Nursing/pumping breaks? Part-time work? Phase back-to-full-work load slowly over a few months? Telecommute? Compressed work weeks?

Where will nursing/pumping take place? How will milk be stored? Other options?

Productivity: If a woman is working fewer hours, how will job expectations be adjusted to reflect that? If she is working the same number of hours, are special arrangements necessary to cover her responsibilities when she is taking nursing breaks?

Supervisor's needs and concerns:

Different types of jobs lend themselves to different return-to-work plans and raise different concerns for supervisors and managers.

Time and Space: Are there particular times that the supervisor needs the woman to be at her desk, classroom, workspace? How long will pumping continue? If there are several women in the same department nursing babies at the same time, how will schedules be arranged to make sure work gets done through nursing breaks and other special arrangements?

Productivity: Who will arrange for the woman's responsibilities to be covered while she takes nursing breaks (e.g., covering desk, classroom, etc.)? Will the pumping breaks be a distraction from accomplishing work tasks on a daily, weekly, or long-term basis? How will pumping impact on the morale of others in the department? If we make special accommodations for this new mother, will others want accommodations as well and how will that impact on morale, productivity, and scheduling?

Nursing mother's needs and concerns:

New mothers have many logistical and broader concerns about the implications of their nursing in the workplace.

Time and space: Is there a designated pumping space available to use every day? Is that space close enough to the workspace to be able to make a "round trip" and pump during the break? Where will breast milk be stored each day? Can breaks be taken at the same time each day? If the baby is in on-site or near-site day care, can the mother nurse the baby directly during the day?

Productivity: How will pumping impact on the morale of co-workers? Will co-workers resent her taking time to pump, telecommute, phase back into work, etc.? Will working from home, fewer hours, different hours change the mother's relationship with the department and/or colleagues and/or clients?

Mothers who plan to return to work and continue to breastfeed should be aware of both their company's policies and the possibilities of breastfeeding while working. There is no reason for the workplace to be the one place where "breast is best" is ignored.

Below are tables that can be used by mothers wishing to return to work and their supervisors to avoid problems and pitfalls.

Naomi Bromberg Bar-Yam, Ph.D., has been teaching, writing, and researching in many areas of perinatal health for thirteen years, including breastfeeding, prenatal testing, and work and the family. She lives in the Boston area with her husband and four children.

In this study of WIC, the federal program (officially named the Special Supplemental Nutrition Program for Women, Infants, and Children), founded in 1972 to address the nutritional needs among low-income women and children, the author sees both hope from what has been accomplished and a potential for further development.

Chapter 10

WIC: Promoting Breastfeeding in a Bottle-feeding culture

Brenda Dobson, M.S., R.D., L.D.

The nutritional, economic, and psychological benefits of breastfeeding are so great that you might expect all families to choose breastfeeding. Breastfeeding seems particularly important for families with limited incomes who may also experience disadvantages due to lack of education and lack of support systems for parenting and healthcare. However, almost half of the formula purchased in this country is purchased for low-income families using WIC funds. In fiscal year 1996, WIC spent $620 million on infant formula (after a rebate savings of $1.2 billion). How can it be that your tax dollars support formula-feeding for a population that stands to benefit greatly from breastfeeding?

THE BEGINNING OF WIC

The federal government established the WIC program (officially named the Special Supplemental Nutritional Program for Women, Infants, and Children) in 1972 to address nutritional needs among low-income women and children that threatened their health and led to higher medical costs. WIC participants receive supplemental foods like eggs, cheese, milk, iron-fortified cereal, vitamin C–rich juices, dried beans and peas, and infant formula.

They also receive nutrition education and referrals for ongoing healthcare and other needed social services. One of the most effective of all federal programs, WIC helps assure normal childhood growth, reduces anemia, increases immunization rates, increases birth weights, and improves the quality of participant diets. Serving over 7.4 million women, infants, and children, WIC is one of the

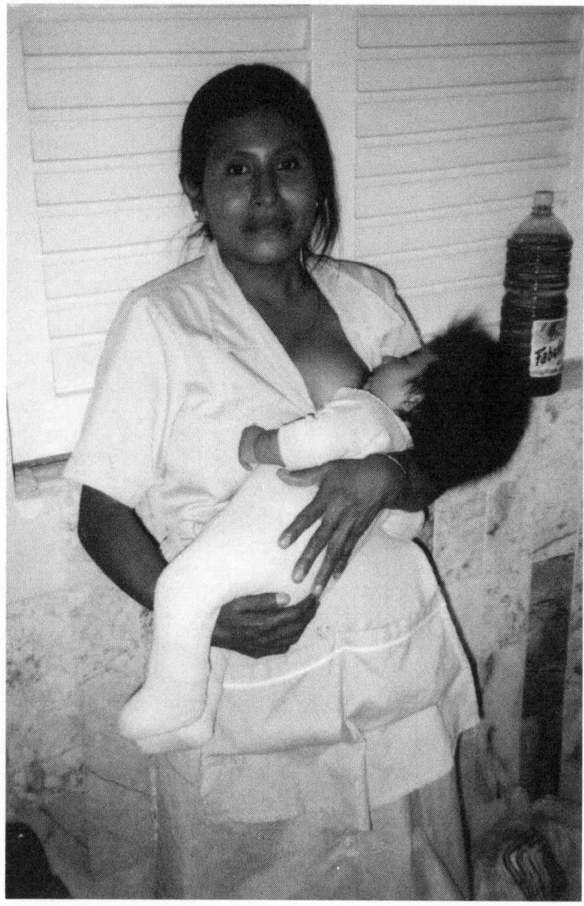

Because of lack of support in the workplace, many employed WIC mothers cease breastfeeding on their return to work following the birth of their babies. However, with guidance from social workers, a mother can learn to juggle the demands of the workplace with breastfeeding her baby.

country's largest, most successful, and most cost-effective nutrition programs. But is WIC really a success if most of the babies served by WIC are not breastfed?

At WIC's beginning, only twenty-five percent of babies were breastfed at birth. Bottle-fed babies started out on infant formula, but often switched to whole cow's milk by six months of age or even earlier. High anemia rates in babies and toddlers resulted. The new WIC program aimed to improve the iron status of low-income infants by promoting breastfeeding and providing commercial iron-fortified formula for babies who were not breastfed. Unfortunately, few efforts were made in the early years to actively promote breastfeeding. Instead early program efforts focused on expanding services across the country, and WIC began to develop a reputation as the formula program for babies.

BREASTFEEDING AS A CLASS ISSUE

Breastfeeding rates increased after 1972, but mostly among women with higher incomes and more education. By 1980, more than half of all mothers breastfed their babies. Breastfeeding rates continued to climb until 1984, when almost 60 percent of all mothers breastfed in-hospital. However, the breastfeeding rates of low-income women, including women participating in WIC, lagged well behind. Like a compatible group in other developed countries, American women with more education and income choose breastfeeding, while poor women and women with less education use formula.

Breastfeeding rates then decreased until the early 1990s. Between 1991 and 1998 breastfeeding rates increased every year. As previously, in-hospital breastfeeding rates are highest among households for mothers who are over the age of thirty, college-educated, non-WIC participants, and who live in the Mountain or Pacific census regions.

Breastfeeding initiation rates are lowest among black infants, mothers less than twenty years old, those living in the East South Central census region, and WIC participants. However, there were increased rates in all demographic categories between 1990 and 1998. In fact the groups with the lowest breastfeeding rates (including WIC) were among the groups with the largest increases. Something must be happening in WIC to make such a difference. Breastfeeding has not been the "normal" or expected feeding choice for low-income families. Can WIC, or anyone else, continue to change these patterns of infant feeding? What are the obstacles faced by low-income families and by WIC?

LACK OF INFORMATION

Sometimes the reasons for not breastfeeding are related to lack of information. This is one area to which WIC devoted much time and energy in the late 1980s and early 1990s. Breastfeeding advocates from within and outside WIC programs strengthened the program's breastfeeding efforts through legislative activities. In 1989, WIC programs were required to employ a breastfeeding coordinator, write a plan to promote breastfeeding, and ensure adequate breastfeeding support for mothers.

Unfortunately, no new money was provided for these activities (contrary to popular belief). Instead, eight million dollars of existing funds were earmarked for these purposes (approximately ten dollars for every pregnant and breastfeeding participant). WIC staff, empowered by their personal experiences with breastfeeding (sometimes positive and sometimes not), began to build a knowledge base about breastfeeding promotion and support. Training events were held for staff, and educational materials were written to replace the industry-based materials that were barely disguised advertisements for bottle-feeding with formula. The message that "breast is best" began to be heard more often in WIC clinics around the country.

Many WIC staff learned to use open-ended questions about breastfeeding to keep the door open for more discussions about breastfeeding. And they learned that they must talk about breastfeeding with every pregnant woman. When healthcare workers assume that only certain women are interested in breastfeeding, they reduce or even eliminate opportunities to reach women who don't realize that breastfeeding is an option.

Sometimes healthcare providers themselves are lacking information and miss opportunities to promote breastfeeding. This may be the case when it comes to promoting breastfeeding to adolescent mothers. A recent study reported that race/ethnicity influences decisions to breastfeed among adolescent mothers. Overall, African-American adolescent mothers were significantly less likely to breastfeed compared with Mexican-American and Caucasian adolescent mothers. Of grave concern is the finding that African-American adolescent mothers were the least likely to report receiving encouragement from their mother, partner, friends, and healthcare providers. In fact, one in four of the African-American adolescent mothers in the study chose to bottle-feed because they were advised to do so by their doctor or nurse.

Breastfeeding should be promoted among all adolescent mothers of all race/ethnicity groups unless medically contraindicated. Information about breastfeeding must target the specific needs of each adolescent mother and include key members of her own support system. WIC has been and must continue to be a source of breastfeeding information for adolescent mothers.

Information is a critical first step to choosing new behavior, but just talking about the benefits of breastfeeding isn't enough. It takes more to result in behavior change. Providers must persuade mothers to breastfeed through discussions, video materials about how to breastfeed, and experiences of other women who have breastfed. Even armed with this information, women may still choose not to breastfeed. Something else is needed to effectively move beyond the "breast is best" message to initiating breastfeeding.

LACK OF SUPPORT

Given the low breastfeeding rates in low-income populations, WIC mothers who choose to breastfeed are bucking the trend. Mothers who receive advice to breastfeed from their own mother or other relatives are more likely to breastfeed. Support from the baby's father, friends, and neighbors is also critical for continued breastfeeding. While some mothers don't have any family members or friends who have breastfed, others lack support due to geographical distance from families. Sometimes the most meaningful thing WIC can do is to help a mother identify at least one mother who enjoyed breastfeeding and who is willing to share information and provide support to other mothers.

WIC programs have developed peer counselor programs (loosely molded, in the beginning, after La Leche League), telephone support systems, and buddy programs to fill gaps in support during the prenatal and early postpartum time periods. Other WIC programs make use of existing peer support groups through referrals. And many WIC programs involve the mother's support network in breastfeeding education and find that it makes a positive difference in breastfeeding rates.

Outside sources of support are also critical for new mothers in the first six weeks postpartum, including support from doctors, nurses, and WIC staff. Mothers who receive advice from physicians to breastfeed are more likely to breastfeed than those who do not receive such advice. Women need such support to get past the early learning stages of breastfeeding. Positive feedback through repeated contacts in the early weeks postpartum increases a mother's confidence in her ability to breastfeed and helps get breastfeeding off to a good start.

WIC staff often share victories about mothers who began to breastfeed but had already stopped by the time they returned to WIC. A recent study (the WIC Infant Feeding Practices Study) followed a nationwide sample of nine hundred mothers who participated in WIC while they were pregnant and during their baby's first year. This study paints a picture of what happens in the hospital. Only twenty-nine percent of WIC mothers gave their infants breast milk as the first feeding; sixty percent received formula as the first feeding; and the remaining received sugar water or plain water. Seventy-two percent of WIC babies slept away from their mothers at least for one night during the hospital stay. Ninety-three percent of WIC mothers received a gift package at discharge, which usually contained items that could and often did discourage breastfeeding (such as formula, bottles, and pacifiers). Almost seventy-five percent of WIC mothers reported some breastfeeding problems while in the hospital, and almost one-third of them received no help from the hospital staff.

So, what happens when they go home? Remember that formula supplementation began soon after birth for many WIC babies. During the first five days, one-fourth receive formula supplementation and half receive supplementation within the first sixteen days. By thirteen days of age, one-fourth of WIC babies whose mothers started breastfeeding are weaned; half of WIC mothers stop breastfeeding by the end of the second month. At any given month during the first year of life, only half, or fewer, of WIC mothers breastfeed without supplementing with formula. And we all know that mothers who supplement with formula stop breastfeeding sooner than those who do not supplement.

Lack of support is more than a WIC Issue; it is a community-wide issue. Besides providing accurate information, WIC staff and other breastfeeding advocates must help mothers grow so confident in their breastfeeding management skills that they demand the services and help that they need to keep breastfeeding. That's a big challenge.

PUTTING WIC DOLLARS TO WORK FOR BREASTFEEDING

When $8 million (of existing funds) were earmarked for breastfeeding in 1989, minimum spending requirements were also set for each state WIC program. Although some members of the WIC community argued against this spending requirement, many were pleased to have breastfeeding expenditures recognized as important public health activities. Having a spending requirement also made it easier to "sell" upper management on the need to increase breastfeeding promotion and support services. Within a few years, WIC was spending well above the mandated level. In 1996, WIC spent $45 million, more than double the mandated spending requirement. These expenditures reflect breastfeeding promotion and support services to mothers and infants; the cost of WIC foods for breastfeeding mothers is not included in this figure.

Also beginning in 1989, WIC programs were required by law to purchase formula from the lowest bidder, usually based on a rebate system. These rebates represent significant savings to WIC. In federal fiscal year 1997, $1.3 billion in savings was attributed to rebates. These rebates support the food costs for almost one-third of all WIC participants, making program expansion possible during times of tighter resources. Rebates are cost-effective and a cost saving to taxpayers, allowing WIC to serve more participants who, in turn, improve their health and ultimately reduce Medicaid costs.

Given these rebates, is breastfeeding a WIC infant associated with any economic benefit to WIC or Medicaid? The Colorado WIC Program carefully looked at this question by examining WIC and Medicaid infants who were breastfed during the first six months of life. Substantial economic benefit to breastfeeding was found, with exclusively breastfed infants saving $478 per infant or $160 per infant after consideration of manufacturer's rebates.

These savings reflect both lower WIC and Medicaid costs for the breastfeeding infants. Total WIC food costs for both breastfed mothers and babies were approximately $10 per month lower than the food cost for formula-fed mothers and babies. This modest savings per infant is substantial when applied to the potential number of infants who could be breastfed. Medicaid pharmacy costs were significantly lower for breastfed babies because of significantly lower recurrence rates of ear infections, gastrointestinal illnesses, and upper and lower respiratory illnesses among the breastfeeding infants. Formula-fed infants had twice the rate of recurrences of each illness studied. These results demonstrate that there is economic benefit to helping low-income mothers breastfeed, saving money in two programs supported by taxpayers.

Much attention has been focused on breastfeeding as a means of reducing infection. Its effects in preventing chronic disease and in promoting child development are not as yet recognized or expressed in dollars and cents. However, these benefits contribute significantly to the quality of life for families.

THE CONTINUED PRESENCE OF FORMULA IN WIC

Formula is a continued presence with almost half of WIC infants being bottle-fed from birth. And many WIC mothers start out breastfeeding but stop early, relying on formula until their baby's first birthday. Can WIC provide infant formula in a responsible way? Should WIC require mothers to breastfeed at least until they return to WIC postpartum?

Requiring mothers to breastfeed does not mean that all mothers will be successful. Breastfeeding means acquiring some knowledge and skills. If mothers are forced to breastfeed before coming to WIC to pick up formula checks, there is legitimate concern that some would not get breastfeeding off to a good start. The end result would be poorly managed breastfeeding, and putting babies at risk. Formula-feeding would basically be delayed for a few days or weeks. Mandating a behavior change in this way would not help WIC spread the word about the benefits and joys of breastfeeding.

What about requiring a prescription for formula at WIC? Infant formula is an interesting food; physicians and other healthcare providers talk about prescribing infant formula, yet families can purchase the product of their choice over the counter. Once home, families often switch between products based on advice from family, friends, their physician—and even from WIC (based on the state programs' current rebate agreement).

Requiring prescriptions for healthy babies is an unnecessary barrier to much needed nutrition. Such an approach emphasizes the class issues of breastfeeding and could potentially make formula even more valued or desirable. A more responsible approach regarding formula use in WIC is careful and limited issuance to breastfeeding mothers. Formula should be issued only in the amounts needed, and always with education and counseling about the potential impact of formula supplementation on establishing and maintaining a milk supply. This is responsible practice and protects breastfeeding for mothers and babies.

THE CHANGING FACES OF WIC

Today, many WIC mothers are either employed outside the home or are completing job training as a result of welfare reform. Many states require mothers of young children to return to the workforce soon after a baby's birth or risk having benefits reduced or perhaps discontinued. These work requirements are yet one more obstacle for low-income mothers, especially given the extra challenges they face in finding affordable quality child care.

Many WIC mothers who are employed start breastfeeding but stop before they return to work or soon after they return. This early weaning is often due to lack of support at the workplace. Few businesses accommodate breastfeeding mothers with time or a room to express breast milk for their babies. Sometimes it's the result of inadequate information. Many mothers do not know that they can combine breastfeeding and bottle-feeding. For most women there is a workable option somewhere between total breastfeeding (including feeding expressed milk) and exclusive formula feeding. They need help exploring their options and planning for their own situation.

WHAT WORKS BEST IN WIC?

Many state WIC programs developed their breastfeeding promotion and support programs on the run—pushed by the need to do something right away and to meet spending requirements. Some jumped right into breastfeeding promotion, while others started out by getting the support networks into place. This is similar to the chicken and egg story—which should come first? The answer is that it depends on the community and the breastfeeding practices that are already occurring.

Effective breastfeeding promotion programs identify barriers or concerns women have about breastfeeding, and then offer strategies to reduce the barriers and help women see that they can indeed breastfeed. This means providing lots of information and support, one mother at a time. Although similar barriers may exist within population groups, each mother brings her unique perspective and life experience to the discussion. When her individual needs are met, breastfeeding is much more likely to succeed.

Breastfeeding promotion programs need effective support systems and services in place. When promotion is effective and more mothers choose breastfeeding, the community must be ready to provide adequate support. This requires WIC programs to work with, and in, their communities on activities like training the staff, developing or obtaining accurate information sources, providing early postpartum support, and building coalitions to draw a community together around its own issues. The strategies for implementing these activities will and must vary based on community needs and available resources.

Media campaigns like the WIC National Breastfeeding Promotion project (sometimes called the Loving Support project) can play an important role in breastfeeding promotion and support. Based upon social marketing research about WIC participants, the project was designed to increase public awareness and garner support of family, friends, and health professionals to work together in support of breastfeeding mothers. Developed with funds from USDA and launched in 1997, the impact of the project is yet to be evaluated. Full implementation of the campaign using several media channels is costly, limiting its use in this time of tighter resources for WIC.

SUMMARY

In 1997, 50.6 percent of WIC mothers initiated breastfeeding, up from 33.7 percent in 1990. This compares to 64.3 percent of all women initiating breastfeeding in 1998. Significant progress has been made among low-income mothers. A dramatic shift also occurred in the attitudes of WIC staff regarding breastfeeding. Most WIC staff now view breastfeeding promotion as central to the program's mission and actively promote breastfeeding in a variety of creative ways. While some WIC programs do a better job (meaning they use a more comprehensive approach) than others, they are all working to improve breastfeeding promotion and support services.

The WIC program is an adjunct to the healthcare system. WIC identifies individual needs for health and other social services, then connects participants with sources of assistance and service through referrals. Breastfeeding promotion and support services, especially for at-risk mothers and babies, may also be a reason for referral. WIC is just the one part of the healthcare system that must provide quality breastfeeding information and support for mothers and babies. It was never assumed that WIC could provide the full spectrum of breastfeeding promotion and support services in every community. Communities must develop common messages and a shared vision to help all women, not just low-income women, succeed with breastfeeding.

It's easy to become angry about spending your tax dollars for infant formula when breastfeeding is the best choice for healthy mothers and babies. The truth is that while breastfeeding is the ideal choice for mothers and babies, it is not always possible. Some women must choose formula feeding due to substance use or abuse, a few medications that are not compatible with breastfeeding, or medical conditions (such as HIV and AIDS) where breastfeeding is not recommended. For other women, a history of childhood abuse, including sexual abuse, may keep them from choosing breastfeeding until these issues are resolved.

Some WIC mothers will choose to formula-feed, some for reasons that we can understand and some for reasons we cannot. It is hard to counsel mothers to be confident about their ability to breastfeed if they have not seen their family members and friends enjoy breastfeeding. Convincing them that breastfeeding can improve their own health and self-esteem and the health of their children is sometimes not enough when they see barriers in their way. Some of these mothers may choose breastfeeding with their next child; some will never give breastfeeding another thought. But WIC can make a difference in their knowledge about breastfeeding, whether or not they choose to breastfeed this baby.

Although the increasing rates of breastfeeding in WIC are encouraging, WIC mothers are still least likely to breastfeed. WIC can take some credit for recent successes, but cannot stop efforts now. Breastfeeding promotion and support services must continue to be a focus in WIC so that breastfeeding becomes socially acceptable and a valued health behavior for all healthy babies, mothers, and families regardless of income.

Brenda Dobson, M.S., R.D., L.D. is a registered licensed dietician and the WIC Nutrition Services Coordinator for the Iowa WIC Program. She chaired the national WIC breastfeeding promotion committee for five years and was the first dietitian to serve on the International Board of Lactation Consultant Examiners. She has been involved in breastfeeding promotion and coalition-building activities in public health for sixteen years.

This chapter is one of the most important in this book. Armed with the knowledge of legislation that exists affecting breastfeeding, women can ensure that they—and their children—can live in an environment that encourages this important health issue. This chapter includes thorough state-by-state information.

Chapter 11
Breastfeeding and the Law

Elizabeth N. Baldwin, Esq.

As more mothers make the healthy choice to breastfeed their babies, more legal situations arise that involve breastfeeding issues. Some of these cases have resulted in a frenzy of media attention, putting various breastfeeding issues in the limelight. Interestingly, the onslaught of breastfeeding legislation in the United States began when a newspaper reporter was told by a security guard that she could be "cited" if she refused to stop breastfeeding in a mall.

The humorous and informative article that the reporter subsequently wrote about the issue caught the attention of a Florida legislator, who was outraged over the fact that any mother would be told to stop breastfeeding in public. The legislation that resulted caught the media's attention, and thus began the powerful and significant changes that have taken place in the United States to clarify a woman's right to breastfeed in public.

While the press eagerly embraces mothers who are told to stop breastfeeding in public, the newest trend is to focus on those who are harassed for wanting to continue breastfeeding when they return to work. One recent case concerned a mother who was fired for wanting to breastfeed her baby on her duty-free lunch break in her own vehicle. The employer erroneously believed that if an emergency arose, a mother would not be able to stop breastfeeding and return to her duties, as she could if she were just smoking a cigarette.

While cases of breastfeeding in public or in the workplace have caught some media attention, the large majority of actual legal cases are rarely reported to the public. The most common legal matter that involves breastfeeding comes in divorce and family law cases where custody and visitation decisions can seriously affect or jeopardize the breastfeeding relationship. It is not unusual for judges to order lengthy visitations with very young babies.

One tragic case involved an order of immediate twenty-four-hour overnight visitations for a four-month-old baby who had never been apart from its mother for longer than four hours. The judge stated that if the baby showed any distress during the visitation, it would be assumed to be the mother's fault, since she was opposed to overnight visitation, and a change of custody would be considered.

Unfortunately, this type of result occurs because breastfeeding as a custom has skipped several generations, and the legal system may not be educated or aware of its importance, or how the father's bond can be promoted without undue, lengthy separations of the baby from the mother.

OTHER LEGAL ISSUES

Other legal issues involving breastfeeding include jury duty, criminal cases, and social service agency cases. In the media spotlight over the past several years are cases of mothers who were charged with murder or manslaughter when their breastfed babies died after the mothers ingested illegal substances. These mothers were convicted of child endangerment or manslaughter and are currently serving prison sentences.

More recently, the popular media have reported a few cases of breastfeeding mothers who were charged with manslaughter when their babies died of dehydration. Sadly, these mothers were often following the breastfeeding advice that our uninformed society had provided for them, without realizing that this "bottle-feeding advice" could result in their babies failing to thrive. In one case, the mother had had breast reduction surgery as a teen. No one, not even the hospital, told her that she might therefore have serious breastfeeding problems and should be closely monitored, even though such a medical history is a red flag for nursing problems. Such tragic situations highlight the essential nature of accurate breastfeeding information and help for mothers.

THE RIGHT TO BREASTFEED

Many people are confused as to whether a mother has a right to breastfeed her baby. The answer to this question depends on what area of the law we are looking at. For instance, the constitutional right to breastfeed, as recognized in a federal court decision (Dike v. Orange County School Board, 650 F.2d 783 [5th Cir, 1981]), does not apply in family law, criminal law, or social service agency cases. Although the constitutional right to breastfeed may apply to breastfeeding in public or in

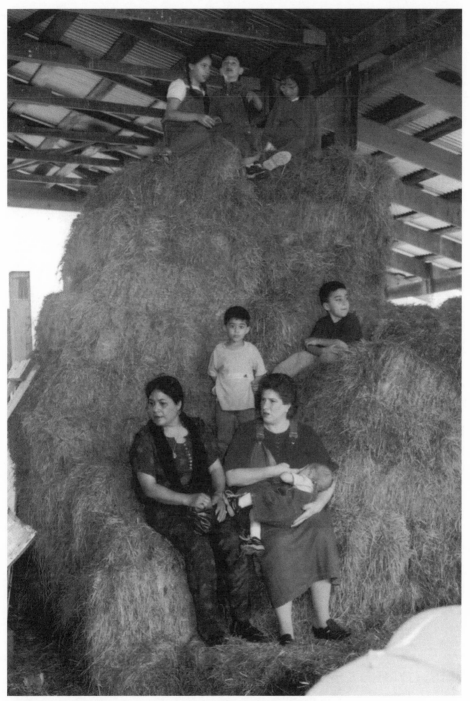

American women traveling in Europe, Asia and Africa are surprised at how commonplace breastfeeding in public is. Here a woman breastfeeds on a hayride outside Bradford.

employment situations, it is still restricted to the public sector, and has not yet been applied to the private sector; even if it were, a balancing of competing interests would be required. There are numerous other legal theories under which one can argue that mothers have a right to breastfeed, but they are not absolute, applicable in all situations, or even understandable to the general public.

Because breastfeeding legislation attempts to clarify a mother's right to breastfeed in certain circumstances, such as in public, there is no need to create theories to support this right. By 1998, nearly one-third of the states had enacted breastfeeding legislation, most of it clarifying or guaranteeing a mother's right to breastfeed in public, and some of it touching on other issues such as the right to express milk at work or the exemption of breastfeeding mothers from jury duty.

BREASTFEEDING IN PUBLIC

Imagine a new mother out in public with her baby for the first time. She finds that her tiny infant is hungry and cannot wait for her to return home to feed. She finds a chair, turns it around, and throws a shawl over her shoulder so no one can see what she is doing. Yet, ironically, this is typically the mother who is asked to leave a store or museum. Although nothing shows, everyone knows she is breastfeeding. It is the idea of someone breastfeeding that seems to offend most people, and the inexperienced breastfeeding mother is more likely to be singled out than the mother who confidently and easily breastfeeds wherever she goes.

Mothers have a constitutional right to breastfeed in public whether there is protective legislation in their state or not. However, the public perception is that breastfeeding is somehow indecent, is an activity that should be hidden, private, and concealed within the home. This public misperception is the reason breastfeeding legislation has been sought and enacted.

What should a mother do if she is asked to stop breastfeeding in public? Many times these conflicts can be resolved by educating the establishment about the importance of breastfeeding and about the current trends in the United States to legislate a woman's right to breastfeed. While being asked to stop breastfeeding can be a very humiliating experience, hopefully the mother will realize that she is doing nothing wrong; on the contrary, she is making a wonderful, healthy choice for herself and her baby.

EMPLOYMENT SITUATIONS

Many new mothers want to breastfeed their baby during the workday or express milk on their breaks. Until recently, many mothers did not know that it was feasible to continue breastfeeding after returning to work. Today, however, more mothers are receiving accurate information and finding quality breast pump equipment available to them.

However, breast pumping is new, and many employers or supervisors are unfamiliar with the process. They not only find it difficult to determine how and where a mother can pump, but they also view breastfeeding as a lifestyle choice and an inconvenience rather than a benefit to the mother, baby, and even the employer as well. Currently, both individual states and the United States Congress are considering legislation to mandate unpaid break time for expressing milk, and to encourage employers to support breastfeeding mothers when they return to work. Currently, three states require employers to accommodate breastfeeding mothers when they return to work: Minnesota, Hawaii, and Tennessee. Mothers who are having difficulty with their employers over breastfeeding or pumping on their breaks should try taking an "I'm sure we can work this out" attitude, rather than threatening to sue. Breast pumping will certainly be a normal part of the workday in the future, as our society becomes more educated and baby-friendly.

On the other hand, some mothers may be forced to take legal action against their employers, especially if they are being discriminated against, or if they live in a state without protective legislation. Women who suspect that they may need to file suit against their employer, or who fear they may end up being fired, need legal advice immediately. Civil actions, including discrimination cases, have strict time limits. A lawyer can advise a mother as to how much time she has under the law to initiate legal action, or help her resolve her situation satisfactorily without litigation.

CUSTODY AND VISITATION: FAMILY LAW MATTERS

Parents going through a divorce or separation must consider what is in the best interests of their children in determining how much time the child will spend with each parent. A crucial issue for the breastfeeding mother is how parenting time can be arranged so that the child has enough time to bond with the father and yet is not separated from the mother for long periods. Generally, parents themselves are best equipped to answer these questions, so the courts encourage, and increasingly require, that parents try to settle custody and visitation issues before turning to judicial remedies. Parents can either come to an agreement themselves, work with a trained mediator, or employ attorneys to negotiate a settlement. Settling benefits everyone involved by saving money, reducing court case loads, and giving parents control in determining the outcome.

As a matter of public policy, states want to encourage children to have a close, loving relationship with both parents after they separate. Courts generally will not allow one parent to unilaterally decide whom the children will bond with or how they will be raised. They want both parents to be involved and to make decisions together as to how they will raise their children. Generally, the courts may recognize that breastfeeding is best, but they will not sacrifice the child's bond with the father so that the child can continue to be breastfed. It is important for mothers to show how the child can continue to breastfeed and, at the same time, have a meaningful relationship with the father. Usually this involves providing for frequent contact with the father without lengthy separations from the mother. Courts should never have to choose between breastfeeding and the father's bond; both are important, and both interests can be protected.

In the United States, many courts consider both parents to be equal with respect to child custody. However, factors such as who is the primary caretaker, or which parent the child is most attached to, may still be considered in determining custody. More and more states are looking at other factors, such as who will provide better access to the other parent, or will help the child, or want to spend time with the non-residential parent. Thus, a parent who is trying to keep a child from the other parent may actually be undermining his or her own case.

Breastfeeding may appear to pose difficulties in establishing parenting time with the father. Standard visitation in many areas, which may be every other weekend, could adversely affect or even terminate the mother's breastfeeding relationship with a young child. Standard summer visitation, of weeks or months without contact with the other parent, can cause such emotional distress as to affect the well-being of these children for the rest of their lives. The best chance of avoiding such standard orders is to provide sensible and practical alternatives to such lengthy separations.

Preparing a specific and detailed parenting time plan is an excellent way of presenting alternatives to standard visitation. Clearly, the parents are in a better position to fashion such a plan than a stranger would be. Plans should be realistic, providing for the greatest amount of time the child can tolerate away from the breastfeeding mother rather than the minimum. Consider that it is rare for any court to postpone overnight visitation past age two. Visitation time should be gradually increased toward the desired goal.

JURY DUTY

The long hours that a mother might spend in a trial as a juror could certainly disrupt the breastfeeding relationship, yet many courts will not make allowances for breastfeeding mothers and do not understand that theirs is a health choice that should be encouraged.

Mothers who are called for jury duty should first determine if they are exempt for any reason. Very few states exempt breastfeeding mothers. Some states may exempt parents of children under a certain age who are at home. Even if a state has neither of these laws, there may be other exemptions that could apply, such as a hardship exemption. A statement from the baby's doctor that specifies the current recommendations about breastfeeding, addresses relevant medical risks that can be reduced by breastfeeding, and recommends that the mother not be separated from the baby may help. Alternatively, the court could be educated about what the mother would suffer in separations: leaking breasts, engorgement, and mastitis and its accompanying fever. Many judges may not be familiar with pumping procedures that would be required if the mother is apart from the baby.

Children are generally not allowed in courtrooms. Although this rule is not aimed at breastfeeding mothers in particular, they could face sanctions if they bring the baby into the courtroom to feed. If a mother must appear for jury duty, one alternative is to leave the baby in the hallway with a friend or relative and inform the judge of the situation.

SOCIAL SERVICE AGENCIES AND CRIMINAL CASES

The right to rear our children is inconsistent with incarceration! Thus, it is not surprising that a mother's right to breastfeed would not apply in these types of cases. A breastfeeding mother who is separated from her baby because of a criminal matter may not have the right to breastfeed her baby, but may be able to postpone serving her sentence or arrange to express her breast milk to relieve engorgement if she is sent to jail.

While a mother might have a legal right to breastfeed her baby during visitation times, mothers are more successful in resolving these issues in a calm, informative manner than by demanding it as their right. On the rare occasion that breastfeeding is directly raised as an issue, information and education must be provided to everyone concerned. Clearly, there is not much anyone can do to help the breastfeeding mother who is charged with manslaughter when her baby dies after she ingests illegal substances. However, it is not recommended that all mothers with a substance-abuse problem wean. Our society needs to help these mothers through substance-abuse programs that closely monitor the mother and allow her to continue providing her baby with this healthy form of nurture.

Occasionally the issue of breastfeeding arises in social service agency cases. One mother was reported to a social service agency when her baby failed to thrive. The standard "knee-jerk" reaction in our society is to immediately place the baby in foster care rather than to examine whether the baby is failing to thrive, and if so, why. Often, misinformation about, and mismanagement of, breastfeeding has resulted in this dire decision.

A great deal of publicity surrounded a mother who claimed she was charged with child neglect for failing to wean her child at an appropriate age. The negative publicity surrounding this case resulted in mothers erroneously concluding that it was against the law to breastfeed past age three, or that they could be arrested or charged with child abuse if they continued to allow their child to wean naturally. In the case cited, the mother was found guilty of neglect for issues unrelated to breastfeeding, and we are not aware of any court in the United States that has found extended breastfeeding to be abuse or neglect, regardless of the age of the child. While many in our society may be unfamiliar with a child nursing past infancy, it is becoming more widely accepted that it is not only beneficial for the child, but also it allows the child to wean in its own time, as nature intended.

CONCLUSION

Our legal system is only a reflection of society's standards. As our society becomes more baby-friendly, we will see these changes reflected in the courts. Until that time, it is important to provide accurate information for all concerned so that legal decisions can truly look at the best interests of our children.

LEGISLATION

Laws relating to breastfeeding, in general:

Laws that exempt breastfeeding mothers from jury duty:
Idaho, Iowa, Oregon

States that have enacted legislation regarding breastfeeding in public (laws that clarify that breastfeeding is not a crime, or indecent exposure):
Alaska, Illinois, Michigan, New Hampshire, Rhode Island, Virginia, Wisconsin

Laws that affirmatively state a woman has a right to breastfeed:
California, Delaware, Florida, Georgia, Minnesota, Oregon, New Mexico, North Carolina, Utah

Laws that provide a remedy to mothers who are asked to stop breastfeeding:
Connecticut, New Jersey, New York

Laws relating to breastfeeding and employment:

States that conducted demonstration projects to determine the feasibility of adopting breastfeeding support policies for state employees (note that the policies have yet to be implemented):

Florida, Texas

States that provide an incentive to private employers to set up breastfeeding support policies:

Texas

States that encourage all employers to accommodate breastfeeding mothers:

California

States that require all employers to accommodate breastfeeding mothers:

Minnesota, Tennessee.

States that declare it is discrimination to prohibit a breastfeeding mother from expressing milk or treating her differently:

Hawaii

For Further Reading:

You can find a summary of breastfeeding laws in each state on the La Leche League legal web page at http://www.lalecheleague.org/LawBills.html

---

Elizabeth Baldwin, Esq., is an attorney and family mediator in private practice with her husband in Miami, FL. Her practice focuses primarily on breastfeeding issues. She is also a La Leche League leader and a member of L.L.L. International's Professional Advisory Board, Legal Advisory Council. She has published numerous articles on breastfeeding and the law and often speaks at conferences as well as assisting in hundreds of breastfeeding legal cases and providing information to parents, attorneys, and other professionals dealing with these issues.

The Baby-Friendly Hospital Initiative is a worldwide program to encourage and support hospitals and other birth facilities that actively encourage breastfeeding. One of the great unknown scandals in the American health picture is that so few hospitals in the United States have received the Baby-Friendly designation. Following is a description of the program.

Chapter 12
The Baby-Friendly Hospital Initiative

Cynthia Turner-Maffei, M.A., I.B.C.L.C. and Karin Caldwell, Ph.D., R.N.

The Baby-Friendly Hospital Initiative (BFHI) is a global program that recognizes the birth facilities which actively take steps to promote, protect and support breastfeeding. This initiative was created by the United Nations Children's Fund (UNICEF) and the World Health Organization (WHO) in 1991. The UNICEF/WHO *Ten Steps to Successful Breastfeeding* form the central core of the Baby-Friendly Hospital Initiative. Support for the *International Code of Marketing of Breast-milk Substitutes* (the "WHO Code") is imbedded in the Baby-Friendly Hospital Initiative. The thrust to create the BFHI came from the 1990 *Innocenti Declaration*, a product of the conference "Breastfeeding in the 1990s: A Global Initiative." The *Innocenti Declaration* identified four operating targets to be achieved in every nation by the year 1995, including:

1. the establishment of national breastfeeding coordinators
2. the practice of the *Ten Steps to Successful Breastfeeding* by all maternity hospitals and centers
3. the implementation of the WHO Code, and
4. enactment of enforceable laws for protecting the breastfeeding rights of employed women

From the inception of the initiative in 1991 through April 2000, nearly 15,000 hospitals and birth centers in more than 128 countries have received the "Baby-Friendly" designation. The greatest number of designated birth facilities is in the region of East Asia and the Pacific, where there are nearly 9,000 designated facilities, representing more than forty percent of all maternity hospitals and centers in that region. A small number of nations, including the African nations of

Comoros Islands, Eritrea, and Namibia, as well as Oman and the Maldives, have achieved designation of all eligible hospitals and maternity centers.

Tally of BFHI Progress

Region Percentage	Number of Baby-Friendly Hospitals	Estimated of Eligible Hospitals Designated
West & Central Africa	1,258	
12%		
Eastern & Southern Africa	574	17
Latin America & Caribbean	1,273	19
East Asia & The Pacific	8,893	43
South Asia	1,565	22
Middle East & North Africa	783	13
CEE/CIS/Baltics	238	4
Industrialized Countries	261	4
GLOBAL TOTALS	14,845	
22%		

Source: *Nutrition Advisor*, UNICEF, 1999 & 2000.

THE BABY-FRIENDLY HOSPITAL INITIATIVE IN THE UNITED STATES

While thousands of birth facilities worldwide were being designated in the early 1990s, the United States was slow to embrace and adopt the Baby-Friendly Hospital Initiative. Implementation of the BFHI was delayed until results of a feasibility study could be obtained. The feasibility study was conducted by an Expert Work Group convened by the Healthy Mothers/Healthy Babies Coalition with the support of the U.S. Department of Health and Human Services. In 1994, the Expert Work Group published a summary report suggesting that international assessment criteria and processes would need modification for use in the United States. The U.S. Committee for UNICEF sought the technical expertise of Wellstart International in adapting and field-testing the U.S. assessment criteria and process. With the guidance of Wellstart International staff and project field coordinator Minda Lazarov, the tool was tested in 1996 in the assessment of the first U.S. Baby-Friendly hospital, Evergreen Hospital in Kirkland, Washington. In the United States, the term "Baby-Friendly" is a trademark of the U.S. Committee for UNICEF.

Article 7. Health workers

7.1 Health workers should encourage and protect breast-feeding; and those who are concerned in particular with maternal and infant nutrition should make themselves familiar with their responsibilities under this Code, including the information specified in Article 4.2.

7.2 Information provided by manufacturers and distributors to health professionals regarding products within the scope of this Code should be restricted to scientific and factual matters, and such information should not imply or create a belief that bottle-feeding is equivalent or superior to breast-feeding. It should also include the information specified in Article 4.2.

7.3. No financial or material inducements to promote products within the scope of this Code should be offered by manufacturers or distributors to health workers or members of their families, nor should these be accepted by health workers or members of their families.

7.4 Samples of infant formula or other products within the scope of this Code, or of equipment or utensils for their preparation or use, should not be provided to health workers except when necessary for the purpose of professional evaluation or research at the institutional level. Health workers should not give samples of infant formula to pregnant women, mothers of infants and young children, or members of their families.

7.5 Manufacturers and distributors of products within the scope of this Code should disclose to the institution to which a recipient health worker is affiliated any contribution made to him or on his behalf for fellowships, study tours, research grants, attendance at professional conferences, or the like. Similar disclosures should be made by the recipient.

Article 7 of the International Code of Marketing of Breast-milk Substitutes published by the World Health Organization in 1981 reflects the critical role health care workers play in impacting the new mother's choice in breastfeeding. (Reprinted by permission of the World Health Organization)

In 1997, the Healthy Children 2000 Project, a Massachusetts non-profit organization, accepted responsibility for hosting the Initiative until a separate corporation could be established to take responsibility for the U.S. BFHI. That new nonprofit corporation, Baby-Friendly USA, was formed in August 1997. Since the spring of 1997, an additional thirteen hospitals and birth centers have been assessed and designated, raising the U.S. total to fourteen designated facilities.

Currently, more than fifty U.S. hospitals have committed to implementation of the *Ten Steps to Successful Breastfeeding* through the Baby-Friendly USA Certificate of Intent program. In order to receive a Certificate of Intent, U.S. birth facilities may submit to Baby-Friendly USA a completed Self-Appraisal Tool, together with a letter of support from a chief operating officer, and an annual fee. Once birth facilities join the Certificate of Intent program, technical assistance is available from Baby-Friendly USA staff. A time line for preparing for assessment is developed by each facility's staff. When the facility feels ready, staff may request an assessment visit.

The on-site assessment is conducted by a team of outside assessors who interview staff, pregnant and postpartum mothers, administrators; observe births and staff working with mothers; and review documentation including policies, curricula, and educational materials. In the United States, results of the on-site assessment are submitted to an External Review Board of experts in the field of lactation. The summary and recommendations of the on-site team are deliberated by the External Review Board, which makes the final designation decision.

Birth facilities are encouraged to contact their national authority for the Baby-Friendly Hospital Initiative to obtain an information packet, including the Self-Appraisal Tool. This document can serve as a guide in identifying positive aspects of current breastfeeding policies and practices, as well as identifying those of concern.

In the United States: Baby-Friendly USA
8 Jan Sebastian Way Unit 13
Sandwich, MA 02563
Phone (508) 888-8044 fax (508) 888-8050
eMail: bfusa@altavista.net
Webpage: http://www.aboutus.com/a100/bfusa

International information:
Advisor, Infant Feeding and Care
Nutrition Section
UNICEF
3 United Nations Plaza
New York, NY 10017
fax (212) 824-6465

All of the world's Baby-Friendly hospitals and maternity centers are to be commended. The question they have been asked is "Who will speak and act for the health of the baby?" They have answered, "We will!"

For further information about the Baby-Friendly Hospital Initiative, contact:

TEN STEPS TO SUCCESSFUL BREAST-FEEDING

Every facility providing maternity services and care for newborn infants should:

1. Have a written breast-feeding policy that is routinely communicated to all healthcare staff.
2. Train all healthcare staff in skills necessary to implement this policy.
3. Inform all pregnant women about the benefits and management of breast-feeding.
4. Help mothers initiate breast-feeding within a half-hour of birth.*
5. Show mothers how to breast-feed, and how to maintain lactation, even if they should be separated from their infants.
6. Give newborn infants no food or drink other than breast milk, unless medically indicated.
7. Practice rooming-in—allow mothers and infants to remain together—24 hours a day.
8. Encourage breast-feeding on demand.
9. Give no artificial teats or pacifiers (also called dummies or soothers) to breast-feeding infants.
10. Foster the establishment of breast-feeding support groups and refer mothers to them on discharge from the hospital or clinic.

*In the U.S., this step has been changed to read "within the first hour of birth."
Source: World Health Organization, 1989.

Cynthia Turner-Maffei M.A., I.B.C.L.C, is the National Coordinator of Baby-Friendly USA. A faculty member of Healthy Children 2000, he is also a member of breastfeeding coalitions on the local, state, and national level, including the United States Breastfeeding Committee. She is the author of a number of publications including *The Curriculum in Support of the Ten Steps to Successful Breastfeeding.*

Karin Caldwell, Ph.D., R.N., is an internationally recognized leader in the field of breastfeeding and human lactation. She is a member of the United States Breastfeeding Committee, convener of Baby-Friendly USA, the implementer of the UNICEF/WHO Baby-Friendly Hospital Initiative in the United States, Chair of the National Healthy Mothers, Healthy Babies Breastfeeding Committee, and Leader of the Eisenhower Foundation annual international delegation on breastfeeding and human lactation.

Section Four

Parenting Issues

Attachment parenting, one of the major philosophical movements in parenting today, ensures that the breastfeeding infant remains close not only to its mother but also to its other parent. Here, in this chapter, some of the major basics of the movement are discussed.

Chapter 13
Attachment Parenting

Katie Allison Granju

Being a new parent today can be confusing and disorienting. From the moment a woman discovers she is pregnant, the information and decision-making overload begins: Will the baby be circumcised or not? Breast or bottle? How much should we hold him? Is it true we should let him cry himself to sleep? What about a schedule? When should I return to my job?

A visit to the local bookstore can leave a parent feeling even more overwhelmed. Childcare guides, often written by male doctors or other "authority figures," generally encourage mothers to ignore their own baby's unique cues in favor of some type of externally imposed list of dos and don'ts.

Although women constantly hear the mantra "breastfeeding is best," they are at the same time assaulted by massive advertising from the billion-dollar pharmaceutical industry which produces infant formula, flooding the media with messages designed to convince women that breastfeeding is difficult, constraining, and not really that important.

Additionally, the modern workplace makes it nearly impossible for mothers and fathers of young children to meet their children's attachment needs while still remaining productive, self-actualized adults. The result of all this? A society full of new parents who feel conflicted and underconfident in their ability to handle what should be the most natural roles in the world: mother and father.

LISTENING TO THE BABY

It doesn't have to be like this! If they will only listen to what they have to say, babies themselves can help to gently guide new parents into a relaxed, fulfilling parenting style that works to the mutual benefit of both parent and child. "But my baby can't talk," a parent may say. Actually, a baby does speak in a language parents understand best. When a just-fed baby begins to nuzzle at his mother's chest, he is telling his mother to bring him to her breast and feed him again, no matter what she may have heard about how often an infant should nurse.

When a young child cries when he is put down to sleep in his beautifully appointed nursery, but seems content and calm when he is held, he is letting his parents know that the most restful place for him to be is nestled beside them in their bed, even if the latest parenting magazine article says that bed-sharing will promote poor sleep habits.

When a toddler clings fearfully when pushed to be more independent, but blossoms into self-assured exploration when allowed to meet the world at his own highly individual pace, he is articulating his need for his parents' continued physical presence. Parents who listen for and validate their own child's cues in this way, rather than making parenting decisions based on societal expectations, other people's opinions, or by the book, are practicing a style of nurturing called "attachment parenting."

ATTACHMENT PARENTING

More and more evidence shows what parents have known instinctively since time immemorial: A secure parent-child attachment in the early years of a child's life lays the foundation for optimal mental, physical, and emotional development throughout childhood and beyond.

Attachment parenting provides the best context in which this important and enriching family bonding can take place. By employing certain hands-on, responsive parenting practices, as well as by interacting with each baby as an individual worthy of respect and dignity, parents can both empower themselves in their roles and develop a strong and loving attachment with their children. Advocates of attachment parenting have identified a variety of ways in which mothers and fathers can utilize the attachment parenting style in their day-to-day lives. These include:

- Minimal parent-baby separation
- Speedy and responsive attention to the baby's signals
- Breastfeeding according to the baby's cues rather than a schedule
- Carrying the baby in a cloth carrier and ensuring frequent skin-to-skin contact
- Sleeping with or very near the baby at night
- Breastfeeding well past the first year

- "Natural weaning" in which the child's needs are respected during the weaning process
- Respect for the baby's unique developmental timetable without pressure for him to become independent before he is ready

Although a complete overview of the concept of attachment parenting can be found in my book *Attachment Parenting* (New York: Pocket, 1999), we will here limit ourselves to a discussion of several of the most basic elements of this special parenting philosophy: breastfeeding, sleep sharing, and carrying the baby.

BREASTFEEDING ON CUE

As the centerpiece of the attachment parenting style, breastfeeding on cue plays an integral role in developing a healthy bond between parent and child. In addition to the critically important health-promoting aspects of breastfeeding, this most natural form of mother–child interaction also enhances a mother's ability to understand and respond to her baby and, in turn, her child's ability to trust her to meet his needs. While it is certainly possible for a bottle-feeding mother to nurture and care for her child, she is without the aid of the biological tie that holds a nursing couple together. It is believed that the hormones that are released into the body of a lactating mammal actually promote maternal behavior toward young offspring. This serves as important support for underconfident, first-time mothers.

Many breastfeeding mothers consider the first year or so of breastfeeding a type of fourth stage of pregnancy during which their babies are still totally dependent on their bodies to nourish and sustain them. And breastfed babies look to their mothers for more than just optimal nutrition. As Sharon Heller, Ph.D., writes in her book, *The Vital Touch: How Intimate Contact with Your Baby Leads to Happier, Healthier Development*, "The arms of the sensitive mother invite. When the world looms too large, too loud, too bright, too cold, the infant knows that she will be enveloped in a warm, protective embrace. This gives the baby a clear message: 'You are safe. You are loved. You are loveable.' And so the infant relaxes, secure against the world." Anyone who has ever seen the look of bliss that comes over a breastfed baby when he is able to calm himself at his mother's breast will not question the central role breastfeeding plays in an infant's healthy emotional development.

The bottle-fed baby, when faced with the same moments of need, can be shortchanged, as can his mother. The bottle-fed infant is hardwired from birth to breastfeeding in short, frequent intervals just like his breastfed counterpart. He may instinctively long to nurse at his mother's breast when he is hungry, tired, wet,

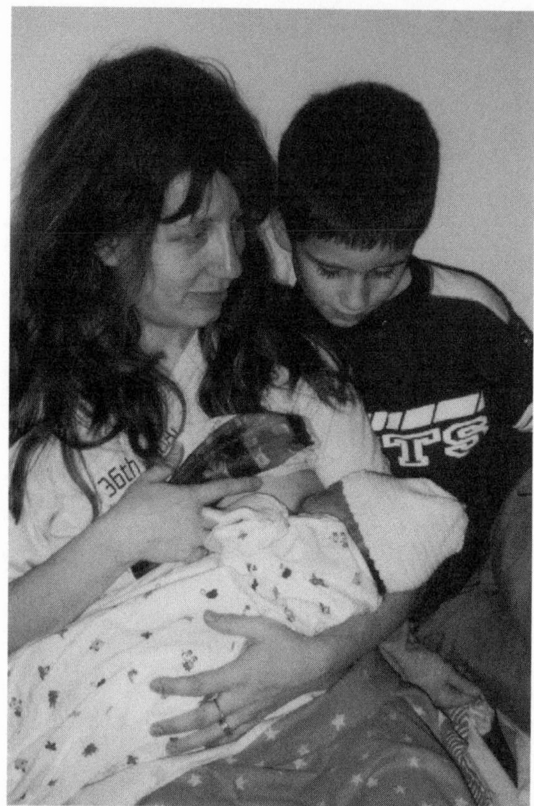

Children in attachment families grow up accustomed to breastfeeding in public as it is a natural way to soothe or feed a child no matter where the family may be.

frightened or over-stimulated. When he fusses, however, his mother is unable to easily know what he needs because she lacks the hormonal breastfeeding connection.

She may offer a hard plastic bottle and nipple, full of synthetic milk, and although this may minimally satisfy his nutritional requirements, his other needs are left unmet. Once he finishes the bottle, she may try jiggling him, rocking him, even giving him a plastic pacifier to suck, but both mother and baby are left without the benefit of the most dependable nurturing tool available: the breastfeeding relationship. Many women who have abandoned breastfeeding too early or who never put their baby to breast at all report strong feelings of sadness and defensiveness regarding their loss of this special tie with their baby.

THE FAMILY BED

Whether a woman breastfeeds or bottle-feeds, however, she, her partner, and her child can utilize other attachment parenting practices in order to reap the benefits of a close and loving family and a well-bonded, trusting baby. Perhaps the most popular of these is family sleep sharing, a practice as old as human families.

All over the world, a wide variety of cultures consider it both normal and necessary for parents to sleep alongside their babies and young children at night.

In the West, however, the foremost rule of family sleep, as promulgated by mainstream parenting experts for the past century, has been that infants and children should never be allowed to sleep with their parents.

This, we've been told, will lead to poor sleep habits, unhealthy dependencies, ruined marriages, and even infant suffocation. Despite such dire warnings and widespread disapproval of the family bed, a growing number of American parents are challenging conventional wisdom each and every night—with support from a new wave of medical and parenting experts including bestselling pediatrician Dr. William Sears, author of *The Baby Book* (Boston: Little Brown, 1993.) and Tine Thevenin, author of *The Family Bed* (Avery, Pub. 1987) as well as researchers such as Dr. James McKenna of the University of California, Irvine School of Medicine.

Emerging research and anecdotal evidence have demonstrated the many benefits of family sleep-sharing. Scores of busy, modern parents, for whom getting a good night's sleep is critical, have decided that co-sleeping actually provides a sounder sleep for everyone in the household, not to mention happier, more secure children. When a breastfeeding mother is snuggled up next to her baby during the night, she barely has to disturb her own sleep in order to tend to him when he is hungry or needs settling. In this way, everyone's nighttime needs are met with little fuss.

The family bed also provides an increased measure of safety for the littlest family members. Parents who sleep with their infants are acutely attuned to their babies' breathing, movements, and temperature. Perhaps not coincidentally, cultures in which family bedding is the norm have much lower rates of Sudden Infant Death Syndrome (SIDS) than do those (such as ours) in which babies are routinely forced to sleep alone in a separate room.

Parents who do choose to sleep with their children will need, of course, to make some basic preparations, such as making sure that bedding is firm, that there is no gap between the mattress and the frame, and that a bedrail will prevent falls, but families who utilize sleep-sharing as part of the attachment style of parenting say that taking these minimal precautions is well worth the effort.

CONSTANT PRESENCE

Not only does attachment parenting offer mothers and fathers a wonderful solution to nighttime nurturing, but this parenting style also suggests ways in which parents and their young children can both have their unique requirements met during the day. Babies and toddlers have an intense need for their parents' nearly constant physical presence as they take their first tentative steps toward independence. Parents, on the other hand, have certain tasks they must accomplish as they move through their daily routine. By carrying her child in a cloth sling, a parent can keep her child close while retaining her own ability to work, do household chores, or go for walks.

Breastfeeding in a sling is easy and convenient. Parents who wear their babies during the day report feeling more attuned to their babies' moods, cues, and rhythms. And it appears that babies who are kept close to their parents' bodies in a sling are more content. Research has demonstrated that babies carried in a sling cry significantly less than other infants. As with sleep-sharing, although Western parents are only recently learning the many benefits of carrying their infants this way, traditional cultures all over the world have long utilized this attachment parenting tool.

Families who wish to learn more about attachment parenting should be referred to *The Baby Book* by William and Martha Sears or *The Womanly Art of Breastfeeding* from La Leche League International. Many mothers especially enjoy the support that comes from meeting others with similar views at local La Leche League meetings.

There are also many Websites on attachment parenting, including www.attachmentparenting.net. However, the best resource for learning about any baby is that baby himself. By listening and responding to him attentively, a mother will soon discover that the two of them may be the only parenting experts needed

---

Katie Allison Granju is the author of the book *Attachment Parenting* and a well-known freelance writer on parenting and health topics. She has served as a Producer with Moms Online and her work has appeared in numerous publications, both print and on the web. She is the mother of three children.

This thorough discussion of weaning a breastfed baby starts from an anthropological point of view and continues to what might be considered the ideal human age for weaning. The chapter also includes preliminary results from a study of children breastfed for periods that might be considered longer than usual.

Chapter 14
Weaning the Breastfed Baby

Katherine A. Dettwyler, Ph.D.

Among the many questions mothers have about breastfeeding, one that comes up often is "How long should I breastfeed?" Both the American Academy of Pediatrics and the World Health Organization recommend that babies start eating other foods at about 6 months of age, and most babies will show interest in what other people are eating by this age. How long, then, should breast milk continue to be a part of a baby's diet, and breastfeeding a part of his relationship with his mother?

The American Academy of Pediatrics' 1997 policy statement on "Breastfeeding and the Use of Human Milk" states: "It is recommended that breastfeeding continue for at least twelve months, and thereafter for as long as mutually desired." In other words, mothers should think of one year of breastfeeding as being the minimum goal and after one year they should continue to breastfeed as long as both they and their child want to.

Since 1979, the World Health Organization has recommended that all children, not just those living in poverty or in Third World conditions, should be exclusively breastfed for four to six months, and then "should continue to be breastfed for up to two years or beyond, while receiving nutritionally adequate and safe complementary foods." In other words, mothers should think of two years of breastfeeding as being the minimum goal. Former U.S. Surgeon General Antonia C. Novello wrote in 1990, "It's the lucky baby, I feel, who continues to nurse until he's two."

Another way to address this question is to ask "Is age at weaning in other primates (our closest relatives among the mammals) related to the way they grow and develop, instead of cultural beliefs, as is the case with humans?" My own research has addressed this question. Studies of nonhuman primates offer different estimates of the natural age for weaning.

PRIMATES

First, large-bodied primates wean their offspring some months after the young have quadrupled their birth weight. In modern humans, this weight milestone is passed at two-and-a-half to three years of age.

Second, primate babies tend to be weaned when they have attained about one-third of their adult weight; humans reach this level between four and seven years of age.

Third, primates wean their offspring around the time their first permanent molars erupt; this occurs at five and a half to six years in modern humans.

Fourth, in chimpanzees and gorillas, breastfeeding usually lasts about six times as long as gestation. On this basis, human babies would be weaned at about four and a half years.

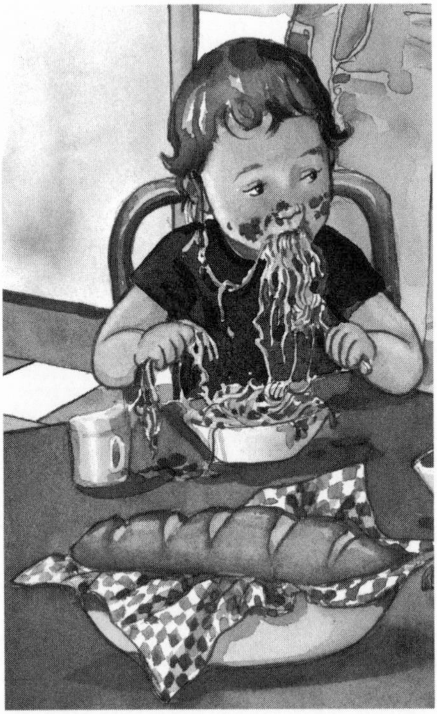

There is no right or wrong time to wean a child. Illustration by Marcy Dunn Ramsey, from *I Was Born To Be a Sister* by permission of Dia L. Michels.

Age at weaning is also related to age at first reproduction in the nonhuman primates. For humans, with first reproduction between twelve and twenty years of age, the predicted age at weaning using this formula ranges from just under four years to over six years of age.

These and other projections suggest that somewhat more than two-and-a-half years is the physiological or "natural" minimum duration of breastfeeding for humans, and seven years approximately the maximum. The high end of this range, six to seven years, closely matches both the completion of human brain growth and the maturation of many components of the child's immune system.

TRADITIONAL CULTURES

Around the world, women in traditional (nonindustrialized) cultures breastfeed their children for three, four, five years, or longer. Research done before the widespread promotion of infant formula found two-and-eight-tenths years as the median length of breastfeeding in a sample of sixty-six such cultures.

Some children in the United States also nurse for several years. Since 1997, I have been conducting research on U.S. children who nursed longer than three years. Of the more than 1,500 children in the sample so far, most breastfed for three to five years, with a range of three to nine years, and an average weaning age of four and two-tenths years

Sadly, because of fear of criticism, many women do not tell their friends, relatives, or neighbors, or even their pediatricians, that they are nursing children of these ages, so it seems less common than it truly is.

Why would anyone breastfeed a child for several years or longer? Contrary to common media depictions of breastfeeding as being painful or a hassle, most women find breastfeeding to be convenient, enjoyable, and empowering.

Mothers of newborns know that breastfeeding is easier, cheaper, and less time-consuming than preparing bottles. Breast milk is always available, can't be contaminated, is the right temperature, and contains myriad nutritional and immunological benefits for the baby. Mothers of nursing toddlers know that breast milk continues to provide the best nutrition available and continues to provide immunological protection, as well as being one of the very best ways to calm and comfort a scared, frustrated, or hurt child. Even small amounts of breast milk can be an important part of the child's diet.

TERRIBLE TWOS?

Although no formal research has been conducted on this topic, mothers who nursed through the second year of their child's life and beyond may say that the "terrible twos" didn't happen to them, they had "terrific twos."

The breastfeeding relationship continues to change as the child gets older and is able to talk to the mother about the importance of breastfeeding in his or her life. Mothers who go back to work and pump breast milk for their infants don't have to pump for the entire time they breastfeed.

By the end of the first year, children can have water or juice with their meals during the work day and continue to breastfeed the rest of the time (mornings, evenings, weekends).

Every study that includes duration of breastfeeding as a variable shows that, up to the study limits of two years, the longer the child is nursed, the better his health and cognitive development. As yet, there has been no research comparing the health of children breastfed longer than two years to those breastfed for only two years.

Although current research cannot claim that there are health and cognitive benefits to nursing beyond two years, it does not support the claim that the health benefits of breastfeeding drop off before the age of two years. In addition, no studies show any detriment to the child from nursing beyond the age of two years.

"Extended nursing" will not make a child clingy or immature, nor will it lead to a "breast fixation"—quite the contrary. Children who were breastfed until they were three or four years of age have wonderful memories of that special relationship. Parents of children who were breastfed beyond the age of two report that their children are independent, secure, and caring.

BREASTFEEDING PROFITS

The benefits of breastfeeding are like the profits from an oil well—you might get $1,000,000 the first year, $100,000 the second year, and only $10,000 the third, but the oil well continues to be profitable, as does breastfeeding.

Undoubtedly, the first week of breastfeeding is the most important week—some studies have found measurable health benefits for some babies from just one week of breastfeeding, compared to those babies who never get any breast milk. Likewise, the first month of breastfeeding is the most important month, and the first year of breastfeeding is the most important year.

However, it may be during a terrible case of flu at age two, the chicken pox at age three, or a stressful family upheaval at age four that one particular child really needs breastfeeding. Breast milk is constantly changing to meet the needs of the child, and always remains superior to any other form of nutrition available; the nutritional value of breast milk does not decline over time.

There is never a time when the milk from another species, such as a cow, is more appropriate for a human child than human milk. Likewise, there are no solid foods that can provide better or more complete nutrition for a child than human milk. Furthermore, neither cows' milk nor solid foods provide immunological protection for the child against diseases.

THE MOTHER'S HEALTH

Let's not forget the mother's health. Breastfeeding has been shown to reduce the mother's risk for several forms of cancer, including breast cancer. In one study, breastfeeding for sixteen months gave women a one-third to two-thirds reduction in risk of breast cancer compared to women who had never breastfed.

Additionally, the mothering hormones released into the mother's bloodstream during breastfeeding, oxytocin and prolactin, help the mother cope with the stresses and strains of caring for young children. These are as important, if not more important, for the mother of a two- or three-year-old as they are for the mother of a newborn.

EASING THE ENDING

When it comes time to bring the breastfeeding relationship to an end, there are a number of things a mother can do to make the experience easier for both her child and herself. Take cues from the child's behavior and let these cues lead the weaning process, even if the mother encourages it along the way. Gradual weaning is always preferable to abrupt weaning. Breastfeeding is a significant and complex part of the child's life; it is much more than simply nutrition. No mother should try to make a child "grow up" too fast, or in too many areas of the child's life at one time.

For example, mothers should not plan weaning for the same month(s) as toilet training or a move to a new house or school.

The mother should talk about weaning with the child, no matter how old or young he is. And the mother should be confident that she has given the child an irreplaceable advantage in life, a life in which a few short months or years of breastfeeding are over all too soon, but will continue to pay dividends throughout their lives.

Katherine A. Dettwyler, Ph.D. is an Associate Professor of Anthropology and Nutrition at Texas A&M University. She is the author of *Dancing Skeletons: Life and Death in West Africa,* which recounts tales of her fieldwork on child health in Mali. *Dancing Skeletons* was awarded the 1995 Margaret Mead Award from the American Anthropological Association and the Society for Applied Anthropology. She is also the co-editor of *Breastfeeding: Biocultural Perspectives,* which includes her own two chapters, "Beauty and the Breast: The Cultural Context of Breastfeeding in the United States," and "A Time to Wean: The Hominid Blueprint for a Natural Age of Weaning in Modern Human Populations."

In most parts of the world, parents and children sleep together in happiness and comfort. It is only in Western society, and only fairly recently, that this is not the case. In this chapter, a leading expert on the family bed provides a thorough discussion of night feeding's advantages to all.

Chapter 15
Night Feeding and the Family Bed

By James J. McKenna, Ph.D.

In a world where people can fly from New York to Paris in six hours, where stocks can be traded with the click of a computer mouse, and film can be developed in less than sixty minutes, the twenty-four-hour demands of a new baby can be overwhelmingly relentless. Even after the evening news is over and the dishwasher has been clicked on, a baby may have no clue that the day is over.

While the rest of the family is winding down, a baby may just be catching his second wind. One technique for managing nighttime routines is for parents to take their baby to bed with them. In our Western society, however, this advice may upset as many people as it comforts.

PARENT–INFANT CO-SLEEPING IN THE FORM OF BED-SHARING

For the past one hundred years in most cultures in the United States, infants have been expected to sleep alone in their cribs from a young age, and parents have been advised to discourage any intrusions into "Mommy's and Daddy's bed." Conventional wisdom has asserted that the family bed is a threat to our culture's ideals of independence and self-reliance, although this contention is completely false as recent studies reveal.

Virtually all laboratory research on sleep in human infants simply assumes that the normal and desirable environment for sleep is a solitary crib in a dark, quiet room far removed from the parents' bed. Mother–infant co-sleeping remains the most appropriate biological and psychological contact for infant and parent sleep, if infant biology and needs are considered first and before recent cultural values

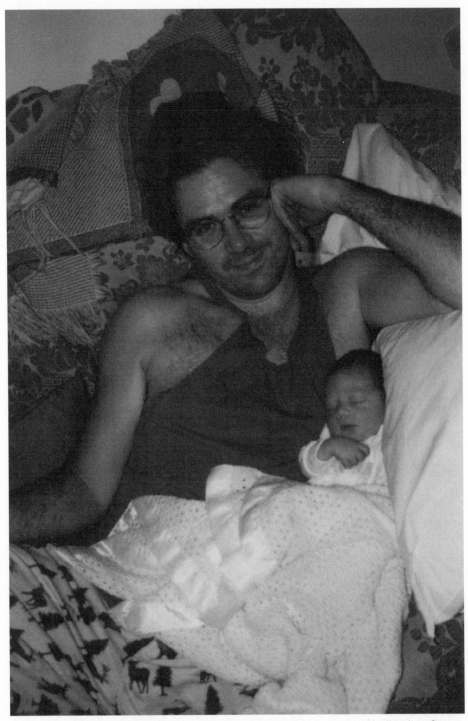

When families sleep together, fathers, too, are part of the nighttime routine with all its benefits to the entire family.

and innovations. Research in the area of infant sleeping arrangements has tended to focus not on the needs of the infant, but on the parents'; specifically, on childcare strategies that accommodate parental work schedules and preferences. No long-term studies have ever actually examined the effects of co-sleeping on independence, and admonishments against the family bed are based on cultural preferences rather than scientific evidence.

OTHER CULTURES, OTHER WAYS, OUR WAYS, TOO?

For most contemporary people worldwide, the family bed remains the predominant sleeping arrangement. Since prehistorical times, infants have slept next to one or more caregivers in order to receive adequate amounts of protection, warmth and breastmilk. From an evolutionary perspective, co-sleeping ensured the survival of infants who otherwise would be vulnerable to the elements and to wild predators.

For the breastfeeding mother, the family bed may well be the ideal place for nighttime nursing. Many new parents, exhausted from their unsuccessful attempts to rock, sing, or walk their baby to sleep, have finally resorted to bringing their fussy baby into their bed. These parents will frequently find that their baby soon settles into a contented sleep.

For new mothers, the family bed can ease the trauma of postpartum sleep deprivation. Contrary to popular belief, recent studies indicate that mothers who bed-share with their babies sleep as much, if not more, than do mothers who sleep apart from their infants. Babies who sleep alone must cry loudly enough to wake the parents, who are sleeping a room or several rooms away.

In comparison, it appears that bed-sharing, breastfeeding babies cry much less frequently and spend less time awake. Babies who share sleep with their mothers tend to nurse more frequently than if they sleep alone, and studies tell us that more frequent infant feedings reduce crying duration, thereby contributing to energy conservation and calm wakefulness.

Consistent with these findings, another study demonstrates that infants who bed-share with their mothers rarely cry when they are ready to nurse. To parents who had expected to get up two to three times a night to feed their baby, being able to breastfeed during the night (without ever leaving the warm comfort of bed) will come as a welcome surprise. When the baby wakes, the mother can simply roll over and nurse. Many mothers will drift back to sleep while the baby breastfeeds. When the baby has finished feeding, he or she will also fall back to sleep.

INCREASED BREASTFEEDING

While it is not known exactly why routine bed-sharing promotes increased breastfeeding, there is research that suggests that breastfed babies are responding to their mothers' unique smell. By two weeks of age, breastfed infants prefer to keep their heads turned toward odor from their mothers' breast. Consistent with the hypothesis of some sort of sensory bridge between bed-sharing infants and their mothers, it has been found that bed-sharing infants remain oriented toward their mothers for much of the night.

This close proximity between infants and mothers, which is facilitated by the co-sleeping environment, would enhance the infant's exposure to olfactory and any other relevant sensory cues from the mother that might promote breastfeeding. This exposure to the mothers' odors during bed-sharing might also have the effect of lowering the infant's arousal/hunger threshold. Studies suggest that infants' bodies have been designed by natural selection to be highly responsive to contact with a primary caregiver, rendering the mother-infant relationship extremely important to a baby's development. Bed-sharing can promote breastfeeding by permitting mothers to respond to the subtle sounds and movements that indicate that their infant is ready to breastfeed.

These frequent nighttime nursings that are common to bed-sharing infants are significant.

Sleep laboratory studies have shown that babies who sleep with their mothers nurse almost twice as much, and for three times as long, as do babies who sleep alone. Human breastmilk is low in fat and protein and relatively high in carbohydrates, especially lactose, which is a key nutrient needed for brain growth. Breastmilk also contains antibodies that help infants fend off disease. Frequent, on-demand feedings benefit babies by increasing daily calories and providing adequate nutrition and weight gain. As infants nurse more regularly, they are also receiving increased numbers of maternal antibodies at a time when their own immunological systems are least efficient. These antibodies may provide breastfeeding, bed-sharing infants increased protection from infectious diseases, some of which are related to sudden infant death syndrome, or SIDS.

BREASTFEEDING AND SIDS

Increased protection from SIDS through breastfeeding is not universally established, but there are several studies that do show it to be protective. There has only been one epidemiological study, however, that has defined breastfeeding categorically (with various cutoffs) and as a continuous variable (months to final weaning and exclusive breastfeeding month equivalents).

This study showed that, for both black and white Americans, the risk of SIDS decreased for every month that a mother breastfed her infant. It may well be that whether or not breastfeeding is protective depends on how many breastfeedings the baby receives.

The sleeping position preferred by infants also influences the risk of SIDS. The supine (on the back) sleeping position has been proven to be critical in reducing SIDS rates among infants worldwide. Studies show that bed-sharing, breastfeeding infants naturally assume a supine sleeping position in order to facilitate access to their mother's breast. Supine infant sleep, perhaps not coincidentally, evolved as part of a larger childcare system: mother–infant co-sleeping with breastfeeding before cigarettes or dangerous drugs or sleeping strictures were invented. Take away the cigarettes and the identifiable dangerous conditions, and whether occurring in New Guinea or Southern California, mother–infant co-sleeping with breastfeeding remains optimal for infant development.

CONTINUAL INTERACTION

Whether nursing or sleeping, throughout the night mothers and babies continually respond to each other's presence. Recent studies indicate that mothers and babies spend more time in the same state of sleep or wakefulness when they sleep together than when they sleep apart. They also experience a significant amount of arousal overlap, in which each partner induces simultaneous arousals of the other, and babies who sleep in a family bed spend less overall time in deep stages of sleep from which arousal is more difficult.

These findings suggest another possible link between co-sleeping and protection against SIDS. Sharing sleep with parents may promote patterns of infant sleep, breathing, and arousal patterns that are most compatible with a baby's developmental vulnerabilities. The frequent arousals experienced by a co-sleeping infant may cause the baby's various subsystems, such as heart and breathing rates, to become better synchronized. These arousals also prevent babies from sleeping too deeply and experiencing an apnea episode (a life-threatening cessation of breathing) before their systems have fully matured.

BENEFITS FOR THE MOTHER

While babies clearly derive health benefits from a co-sleeping, breastfeeding environment, mothers do, too. According to one study, the more frequent nighttime breastfeedings that occur with routine co-sleeping, and the longer duration of these feedings, reveal a nocturnal breastfeeding structure that is consistent with that known to suppress ovulation. Recent studies suggest that frequent nipple contact or sucking combined with relatively short intervals between breastfeedings are required to sustain the high levels of circulating prolactin which are known to suppress ovulation.

Not all mothers who both breastfeed and bed-share, though, will experience this effect. When it does occur, ovulation suppression contributes to the mother's increased iron reserves by delaying the blood loss associated with menstruation, and can prevent her from becoming pregnant again before her baby is ready to be weaned.

AVOIDING DANGERS

Many parents who are considering bed-sharing worry about accidentally rolling over and smothering their infant. Such incidents are extremely rare. Most parents develop a subconscious awareness of their baby's position on the bed and avoid rolling onto that area. In the event that a parent does get too close to the infant, the baby's cries and movements will alert the parents to any danger.

In order to maximize the safety of the sleeping environment, sleep surfaces and structures must be evaluated for safety.

Co-sleeping on soft mattresses, sheepskin, beanbags, waterbeds, or other thick, soft items could result in suffocation. Keep comforters and pillows away from the infant's head, and to prevent overheating; babies shouldn't be blanketed more heavily than the adults—including by sleep suits.

To prevent infants from slipping between the mattress and the bedframe or headboard, fit them tightly at all mattress–frame intersections. Sharing sleep on couches should be avoided, as babies can become trapped against the back of the couch and can fall into a crevice created by the seat cushion.

Parents may be reluctant to bring their baby into bed with them for fear that the infant will fall to the floor. In order to keep infants and small children from rolling out of bed, push the bed firmly against the wall. Bed rails are also available to prevent children from tumbling onto the floor. Alternatively, the mattress can be placed on the floor to eliminate any danger of a fall just as long as the mother is not pushed against a wall or a piece of furniture. Infant deaths have occurred when, unbeknownst to the parents, the mattress has pulled away from the wall, making it possible for an infant's head to get wedged, leading to asphyxiation. If bed rails are used, it is critical that the spacing of the bars does not permit the infant's head to slip between them. Bed rails have not been regulated for safety, as crib slats have. Another option is to place the infant's bassinet or crib within arm's reach; this way, parents can respond to their baby's cues, but the baby is safe from many of the risks associated with bed-sharing.

THE CONS OF BED-SHARING

It is extremely important that mothers who smoke never sleep with their infants. Cigarette smoke is associated with an increased risk of SIDS—even smoke residue on clothing or bed sheets must be avoided. Other reasons to avoid the family bed include parental use of alcohol, drugs, or medications, all of which could impair the ability to respond to the infant in a safe manner.

While it is rare for an adult to overlay, or suffocate, a co-sleeping infant, this tragedy is much more likely to occur if a parent is under the influence of any substance that causes a sedating effect.

TRADITIONAL COMFORT

For millions of years, parents have lulled their babies to sleep by bringing them into the family bed, where they were nursed to sleep and nursed on demand throughout the night. What constitutes a "bed" is, however, highly variable so attention should be given to the specific condition of the bed to make sure that it is safe. No crevices or spaces should exist, for example, into which a squirming baby or toddler could fall. This warm and protective environment remains the norm for most contemporary people worldwide, and sleep laboratory studies have shown that bed-sharing infants breastfeed more frequently and cry less often.

In Western societies, however, parents today are often advised to encourage their child's self-reliance and independence by putting the baby to sleep, alone, in a crib far removed from the parent's bed. To frazzled mothers and fathers who have endured the ritual of listening to their infants frantically "crying it out" down the hall, a return to the traditional family bed can ease nighttime routines and provide peace of mind for both parents and baby.

James J. McKenna, Ph.D., received his undergraduate degree in anthropology from the University of California, Berkeley, his Master's Degree from San Diego State University, and his Ph.D. in Biological Anthropology from the University of Oregon. He is presently Professor of Anthropology at the University of Notre Dame, where he directs the Mother-Baby Behavioral Sleep Center. He is the author of over 130 articles published in medical, anthropology, and psychology journals and is currently writing a book for the wider market on parenting entitled *The Society Who Mistook Their Children for Bats or Why Infants and Children Have Sleep Problems to Solve*.

Section Five

Special Circumstances

As medical science advances beyond what was only dreamed of years ago, more and more premature babies are surviving. Their births—and their futures—bring with them many concerns for their parents. In this sensitive chapter an internationally known doctor discusses issues and ways in which even a premature baby can be ensured the benefits of breastfeeding.

Chapter 16
Breastfeeding the Premature Baby

Marcus Renato de Carvalho, M.D., M.P.H.

Having a premature baby is an undesirable and unpredictable occurrence, which can bring forth disturbing and contradictory feelings. Parents often express anxiety and guilt caused by the fear that they might have done something to cause the premature birth, or that they might have overlooked some important preventive procedure that would keep the child from suffering. These emotions can be greatly increased by the fact that the premature baby is usually separated from the parents and placed in an Intensive Care Unit (ICU). A first step for professionals in helping the parents cope with these emotions is helping the parents acknowledge them and encouraging them to talk about them to health professionals—especially psychologists in charge of offering support to parents of premature babies.

THE CLOSER, THE BETTER

To the parents of a premature baby this so-wanted baby may turn out to be a most frightening image: she is in an incubator—bald, lying under a glass dome, diapered, hooked up to tubes, to a urine collector, and to monitor wires.

Despite the technological setting, the little thing lying there is their baby! She really needs to feel the touch of their hands, to hear their voices and, as soon as it is possible, to be taken in her parents' arms. Remember: It has been widely proven that the physical interaction between the parents and the baby is positively related to fewer respiratory arrests, to a greater weight gain, and to a faster recovery of the neonate. To the mother this interaction will be very comforting, too. It will make her feel useful and it will help her to produce more milk for her baby.

An important thing to keep in mind is that the parents should have free access to their baby in the ICU at all times. In fact, in the ideal situation, the mother and father get to spend the greatest amount of time possible with their infant. In those cases where the mother is released from the hospital before the baby, her subsequent visits to the ICU should be long and frequent. The father can also help a lot during this phase and should be around as often as he can be, interacting with his baby at least once a day.

A SPECIAL DIET

The premature baby was born before his complete intra-uterine maturation could take place and this condition puts him in a risk group. Parents should understand their baby is now quite dependent on the kind of nourishment he will get. In this critical developmental phase, neonatologists, nutritionists, breastfeeding consultants, and the parents should work side by side, so that the best possible nourishment is offered to the baby.

If a health crew is not supportive of using breast milk, it is the duty of health professionals to acquire a second opinion. Parents will be happier and the baby will be healthier if they work with professionals who understand the miracle of breast milk.

The available literature shows that neonatologists find better development rates in premature babies who were offered maternal milk than in those who received industrialized baby formulas from cow's milk. The mother of a premature infant produces milk that is higher in protein and salt concentrations—to mention only two of many elements—which can perfectly meet the premature infant's special needs. Thus, the best food for a baby, whether full-term or premature, is right inside the mother!

IMMUNOLOGICAL TRANSFUSION

The physical contact between the mother and her baby should be promoted because it not only strengthens the bonding between them, but it also facilitates the immunological transference from the mother to the neonate through the cycle "intestines-lungs-mammary glands." In this system of immunological export, the mother involuntarily intakes and breathes antigens (bacteria, viruses, and hospital fungi) and her body produces specific antibodies (immunoglobulins) that will migrate to the mammary glands and will ultimately be transferred to the baby through the milk.

Colostrum

A little before the delivery and for the first three to four days after the baby is born, most women's breasts will start releasing a very special kind of "milk," called colostrum. Colostrum is a thick, yellowish fluid rich in protein, antibodies, and other infection-fighting agents such as leukocytes (white cells). It is easily ingested and has laxative properties that often guard against neonatal jaundice. It also contains hormones, growth components, and many other nutrients that should not be wasted. Even small quantities of this substance—just a few drops—can make a difference in the prevention of necrosing enterocolitis, a frequent intestinal pathology affecting the neonate.

Colostrum is gradually replaced by early, or transitional, milk. Parents are often surprised at the way it looks. It is very plentiful, light, and thin because it is eighty-seven percent water. Within about two weeks of the baby's birth, this early milk is replaced by bluish-white mature milk.

THE METHODS OF FEEDING LOW-WEIGHT BABIES

Depending on her clinical condition, a neonate with a thirty-week gestational age or less can be fed maternal milk through a nasogastric catheter. At the age of thirty to thirty-two weeks, maternal milk may tentatively be fed from a glass, a spoon, or in drops. After thirty-two weeks and a weight of approximately 1,300 grams, breastfeeding is sometimes possible, but it is only after thirty-six weeks and a weight of 1,800 grams that direct feeding becomes more coordinated and, most of the time, feasible.

Kangaroo Care

Depending on the clinical condition of the premature baby, some intensive care nurseries may adopt what is called "kangaroo care," a therapy that enables the recovery of the neonate through the direct nourishment and permanent contact with the mother's body.

The premature infant is put in a special baby bag under the mother's clothes. Feeling the mother's heat, breathing rhythm, and heartbeats, and sucking a little on the mother's breasts, many times day, the baby may recover much faster. However, this system is not right for every infant. Some babies, whose conditions are more serious, will only improve through the high-tech medical procedures and professional care offered in a well-equipped ICU.

The best milk for a premature baby is her mother's! A pre-term baby's mother produces special milk, with higher concentration of proteins, calories, sodium, and lower concentration of lactose than term-milk (thirty-seven- to forty-two-week gestational age). Thus, the mother must be ready: the premature baby's most urgent need is her mother's.

During the time that the baby is in the ICU, whether he is being fed his mother's milk or not, the mother should stimulate her milk production by means of hand or machine expression, making the milk flow. Health professionals, lactation experts, other mothers and friends should be prepared to help the mother who is not able to extract any or enough milk, or to assist when there is breast engorgement. By releasing milk from the breasts several times a day the mother will be ready to breastfeed as soon as the baby is ready.

A MILK RICHER IN FATS

At the end of each breastfeeding session mothers must know they produce a very special kind of milk—the hindmilk. This milk that comes later is much richer in fats than the milk at the beginning of the nursing session. It therefore provides much more energy and is richer in calories, guaranteeing great benefit to the baby.

Since milk at the beginning of a feeding session is different in composition from milk at the end, breastfeeding sessions should begin and continue calmly until each breast is completely emptied and the mother has made the two kinds of milk available to the baby. Mothers should know that it is the continued sucking motion of the baby or the hand or pump expression throughout the session that will stimulate the secretion of a hormone called oxytocin, which will ultimately make hindmilk eject from the breasts. Oxytocin causes the smooth muscles surrounding the lobules to squeeze hindmilk into the breast's ductal system, a process known as "letdown" or "ejection reflex."

When mothers are making the milk flow manually, they should store the hindmilk in a separate sterile container and label it, so that its great nutrients are not wasted and can be offered to the baby later.

RELEASING THE MILK FROM THE BREASTS

The hospital should provide mothers of premature babies with sterile containers where they can store their milk. Breasts do not need any special hygiene. They should be washed thoroughly once a day during the mother's regular bath. The mother's hands and arms should be very clean and dry.

There are several ways of extracting milk from the breasts. Some nursing mothers can do it very well with their hands. Others must do it with a special electric pump. There are several models of pumps. It is important for hospitals and lacta-

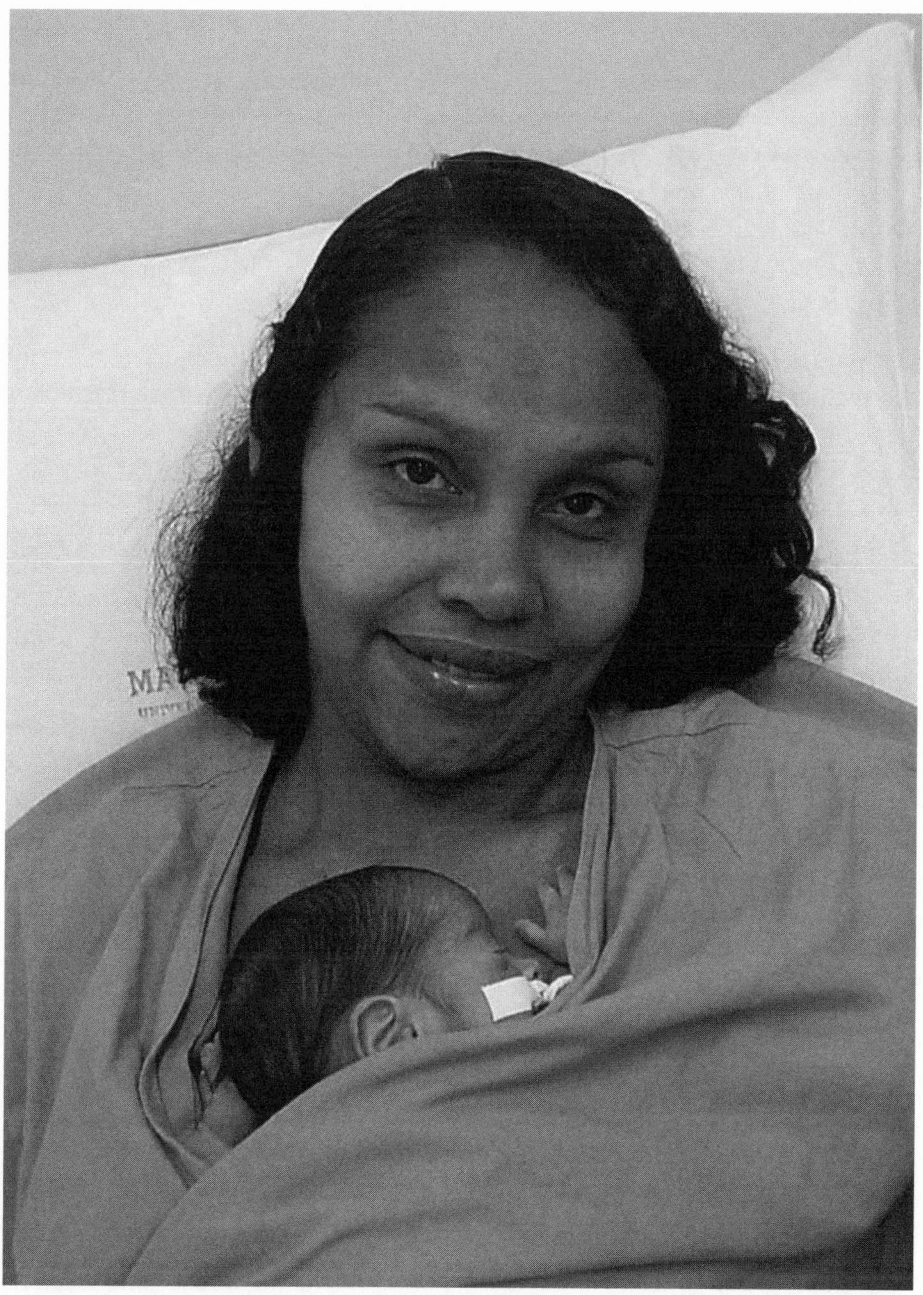

The premature baby generally has difficulty in breastfeeding, and will not be able to suck firmly for more than a few minutes. The mother therefore will need strength and patience; she may need to sit, relaxed and comfortable, in an armchair for more than an hour, cuddling the baby as he tries to feed. A nasogastric catheter can substitute for feeding, if needed. Photograph reproduced with permission of Marcus Renato De Carvalho, M.D.

tion specialists to help mothers find the one that best suits each woman since some may hurt and others might not be very efficient.

Mothers should be encouraged to keep one thing in mind: The fact that it may seem very hard to extract milk at first does not mean that a woman does not have enough milk. Relaxation and comfort, alone or in the company of supporting or professional people, are essential. Some mothers alternate breasts several times during one milking session. Others prefer to empty one breast completely and then start on the other.

Both ways work fine if the mother keeps the final milk in a separate container to feed the baby a more nourishing milk. Remember that the more milk the mother produces, the more milk she will have. During the nursing period a mother should rest, sleep, and eat well and should drink more water than usual. In order to maintain an adequate milk flow, a nursing mother should breastfeed or express her breasts at least six to eight times in twenty-four hours.

There is no special care a nursing mother should take in relation to food and drinks, except for avoiding alcoholic beverages, coffee, tea, and soda that is not caffeine-free. Excessive caffeine consumption by a breastfeeding mother may make her baby fussy and wakeful.

Smoking is not advisable either because it diminishes the production of milk. If the baby is being fed human milk that is not its mother's—a situation which is not ideal—this milk should be pasteurized so that it does not transmit any diseases. Pasteurized human milk is still far better than the baby formulas made of cow's milk.

STORING MILK

Breast milk should be stored in the main section (not the door) of the refrigerator for no longer than twenty-four hours. Milk from different milking sessions of the day can be stored in the same container. After filling the container, it should be closed immediately and labeled with the time and day of the extraction. If the mother wants to store the milk for a longer period of time, it can be placed in the freezer immediately and stored for up to three months.

If the premature baby is in the ICU and the mother is at home, she can transport the milk to the hospital in a box with ice or in a thermal container. The nurse in charge of the ICU should inform the parents of the quantity and frequency of their baby's feeding sessions.

BREASTFEEDING THE PREMATURE BABY

The long-awaited moment when the mother finally breastfeeds her baby may be frustrating at first because the little baby may have difficulty sucking on the breast (on the nipple and around the areola). The mother should try to position the baby the best possible way. A phono-audiologist may perform a motor-oral test with the baby, to evaluate its sucking strength, position of the tongue and lips, and if there seems to be a problem, to stimulate the baby to suck correctly.

Pacifiers and bottles should not be used because they may cause a motor-oral dysfunction "called nipple confusion." Nipple confusion describes how the practice of sucking on a rubber nipple hinders the correct sucking on the mother's breasts.

Mothers of premature babies should be available to spend many hours of the day in the hospital because premature babies have long, and sometimes quite inefficient, breastfeeding sessions. The baby is very fragile and sleeps for long periods and certainly will not be able to suck firmly for more than a few minutes. The mother should be relaxed, and sit in an armchair that can comfortably support her arm and the child. Advise her to try to be confident, no matter how hard it may be. Some hospitals have arrangements so that the mothers of premature babies can stay overnight at least now and then.

The mother should squeeze a little milk into the baby's mouth, so that the baby can feel its taste and smell by pressing the areola between the index finger and thumb, so that the baby can take the nipple. Rubbing the nipple lightly on the baby's cheeks, so that the search and seizing reflex is triggered, often helps. Mothers should not be frustrated if the baby does not suck correctly in the first session.

SUPPLEMENTS

Nature could not foresee the advancements of science and with them the survival of smaller and smaller premature babies. In their intrauterine life they were nourished via blood, through the placenta and umbilical cord. If that nourishment ceases to exist for extremely premature neonates, of very low weight, nourishment administered parenterally may become necessary. Only after some time can such neonates be fed an oral diet.

In some cases it is possible to use a supplemented milk, that is, an insert made of proteins, calcium, phosphorus, sodium, potassium, chlorite, and magnesium that is added to the mother's milk in order to provide extemporaneous neonates with all their special needs.

An even better alternative is supplementing the mother's milk with powdered human milk, produced by means of a dehydrating technique available only in some healthcare centers.

BACK HOME WITH THE PREMATURE BABY

When the premature baby finally comes home it is a time for readaptation for the whole family. The baby may reject the breast at first because he perceives that the environment is different, but this can be overcome—with patience and tenderness. In case the daily weight gain of the baby is not satisfactory, the mother can supplement breastfeeding with the administration of her own milk in drops.

In the beginning the pediatrician or other health professional should assist mother and baby as frequently as every two days or at least once a week. It will help if the mother makes note of the number of times the baby urinates and evacuates each day as well as the color and density of the baby's feces (bowel movements).

When it is time to breastfeed the baby, the mother should do it in a warm place so that the baby can be dressed only in her diaper and can have direct contact with the mother's skin. The mother should hold him as long as she can. No new mother should be embarrassed to ask others to help with the household chores. A new mother's priority is the new baby.

With the right kind of support, many women succeed in breastfeeding their premature babies. The information in this chapter will help. Furthermore, the mother will feel the joy of having her baby's skin touching hers, and the joy of trying to give the best nourishment she can to her baby.

Marcus Renato de Carvalho, MD, M.P.H., is a professor of pediatrics and a breastfeeding consultant in Rio de Janeiro, Brazil. A graduate of the National School of Medicine at the Federal University of Rio de Janeiro, he has worked extensively in the field of social and preventive medicine at the Social Medicine Institute and received advanced training at the National School of Public Health at Fio Cruz. His postgraduate studies include the Lactation Management Education Program given by Wellstart International in San Diego, California. He is internationally known for his studies of breastfeeding and breastmilk substitutes as well as for his many committee memberships and publications. He has also made advertisements telling of the virtues of breast milk which have appeared on Brazilian television. Website: http://www.aleitamento.med.br/

Yes, adopted children can be breastfed and, in cases where breastfeeding has been interrupted for reasons of the mother's or child's health, breastfeeding can be resumed. But it is not easy and it is not always possible. This warm but realistic chapter offers suggestions about how to induce lactation and adjust emotional responses to difficulties.

Chapter 17
Nursing the Adopted Child

Induced Lactation and Relactation

Kathleen G. Auerbach, Ph.D., I.B.C.L.C.

Every breastfeeding relationship is unique for the mother and baby experiencing it. Some situations are more special than others. Relactation (breastfeeding after some period of not breastfeeding the baby) and induced lactation (sometimes called adoptive nursing) are two examples. Why? Because they refer to situations that may seem—at first glance—to make breastfeeding more difficult or impossible to accomplish.

RELACTATION

Relactation generally refers to the resumption of breastfeeding after any delay or interruption of at least a week or more. For example, the mother became ill or injured, had to be hospitalized, and continued breastfeeding was not possible or not practiced. The return to breastfeeding is called relactation, meaning that the mother is seeking to produce milk again although her supply is now extremely low or nonexistent. Or perhaps the mother is well, but the baby is ill or was injured. Relactation may be necessary after the baby returns home.

Or perhaps the mother weaned the baby from the breast fairly early and then decided, perhaps because the baby could not tolerate nonhuman milks, to return to breastfeeding some time later. In the past, relactation also was an issue for many mothers of premature infants because they were not allowed to begin breastfeeding, and no one suggested that they begin breast pumping immediately. Fortunately, this is rarely the case today, when neonatal intensive care nursery staff help the mothers of these tiny babies to begin pumping soon after the baby's birth.

Regardless of the reason for relactating, the key to doing so is frequent, effective nipple stimulation by the baby, with or without the additional assistance of a fully automatic intermittent electric breast pump or hand expression. If the baby's condition is the reason the mother needs to relactate, she may need to use a breast pump to initiate milk production. Ideally, the baby will be returned to the breast as soon as possible. Often, she or he can be encouraged to suckle well and often, if an initially meager supply is supplemented from a device that provides milk at the breast, rather than from a bottle.

Most lactation consultants have such devices and can assist in their use after determining that such a device is appropriate. With such stimulation, it may not be too long before mother and baby are once again a happy breastfeeding couple. However, making a complete milk supply does not always occur. Both parents and professionals should define "success" in terms of getting the baby back to the breast, rather than solely from evidence of milk production.

When estimating how long relactation is likely to take, it is wise to estimate at least twice as long as the baby was off the breast or the mother was not breast-

Myth	**Reality**
It is necessary to be pregnant in order to make milk	Nipple stimulation makes milk. If the baby is put to breast frequently, the mother will make milk.
If a woman has been pregnant before, she will make more milk than if she has never been pregnant.	Reproductive history does not predict how much milk a woman will make; the best predictor of milk production is how frequently and effectively the baby goes to the breast.
If a mother has breastfed at least one birth baby, she will make (more) milk more quickly than if she had never breastfed.	Breastfeeding a previous child does not predict how a new baby will breastfeed or how a mother's body will respond to such stimulation. The only benefit found to occur in mothers who have previously breastfed is a slightly more rapid initiation of milk production, but this does not predict milk volume.
If a mother is already breastfeeding a baby or birth-child, she will make a complete milk supply for the adopted baby in a short time.	The milk a mother makes for a birth-baby or child is geared to that baby, not to the adopted baby. There is no way to guarantee a complete milk supply for the adopted baby.

Myth	Reality
If the birth-child being breastfed already is not yet on solid foods, the mother will make a complete milk supply for both babies.	How the birth-child is breastfeeding does not predict how much milk the mother will make.
Taking hormones is necessary to make milk.	It is not necessary to take hormones in order to make milk. Milk production is stimulated best by the baby suckling the breast frequently and effectively.
Breast pumping will bring in and maintain a milk supply for the adopted baby.	Some mothers find that breast pumping in advance of the adopted baby's arrival helps develop an initial milk supply, but rarely is the mother able to maintain such a milk supply. And, nothing is sadder than seeing milk come in, only to have it disappear before the baby has arrived. If you want to pump, do so after the baby arrives.

feeding. Some mothers are pleasantly surprised when milk production occurs in a shorter period. Worrying about milk production or its evidence will simply make the process more difficult.

INDUCED LACTATION

Induced lactation refers to breastfeeding the adopted infant. Many myths and misunderstandings abound about breastfeeding adopted children. Reviewing these myths and knowing the reality of the situation can help mothers understand what to expect of themselves and their baby if they are thinking about breastfeeding an adopted baby.

The key to adoptive nursing is first getting to know a new child just as the mother would if she gave birth to a baby. I suggest that the mother take the baby to bed when they arrive home from the hospital or adoption agency. She should strip to the waist, leaving the baby's diaper in place. They can then snuggle together under the covers with the baby lying on the mother's chest between her bare breasts. The mother should give the baby a chance to feel and hear her heartbeat and her voice, and to feel her hands as she gently rubs the baby.

If the baby begins to root (look for the breast with his mouth and tongue), the mother should slide him over to one breast and let him explore with his tongue and mouth. If he starts to suckle, she should let him do so. This first contact is not so much a "feeding" as a "hello there" time. If the baby wants to feed later, the mother should use a tube-feeding device so that the baby can suckle the breast (stimulating the body to make milk) while he is receiving nutriment from the tube device. All subsequent feedings should include use of the device as well.

The age of the adopted baby may predict how likely he will go to the breast. Most babies under three months will exhibit a rooting reflex if given the opportunity, even if he has been bottle-fed from birth. Thus, a baby adopted right out of the hospital or shortly after the baby's birth will probably root and latch on to the breast with minimal hesitation.

Babies between three and six months are a little "iffier." Babies adopted from overseas are likely to be in this age group or even older. Often these babies were abandoned shortly after birth and have been primarily bottle-fed. The older they are, the less likely they are to exhibit a rooting response, and the less likely they are to respond to the breast. Sometimes, offering the breast when the baby is sleepy will cause him to respond as if he were younger.

In nearly all cases, babies over six months old cannot be convinced to suckle the breast. Particularly if they have been bottle-fed for many months, they may have no idea what to do. For them, sucking is for a pacifier or a bottle of milk, water, or juice.

Asking such a baby to breastfeed may be asking for more than he or she can be expected to do. The mother must not blame herself. Unlike artificial feeding, breastfeeding is a two-person activity. This requirement that both parties work together is true for all breastfeeding and is most obvious when a mother and her adopted baby are attempting it. A mother can want it with all her being, but if the baby does not know what to do, breastfeeding will not occur. If this happens, the mother should simulate breastfeeding when she is feeding the baby by holding and cuddling this new little person. She should help him to see that his mother is an adult he can trust.

SOME FINAL THOUGHTS

Breastfeeding is a way of enhancing a new baby's psychological attachment to the mother and other family members. It is what I call "milk from the heart." Babies gain a sense of security not only from breastfeeding, but also from the holding and touching and closeness that is enjoyed so naturally when putting the baby to breast. In a relactation situation, this frequent holding and touching does much to encourage the baby to come back to the breast, particularly if many weeks have elapsed since his birth or his last breastfeeding.

It is not possible to predict which adoptive breastfeeding couples will enjoy a small or large milk supply. This depends greatly on two things: the baby's breastfeeding pattern and the mother's body's response to such stimulation. One adoptive mother who achieved a moderate milk supply commented that her baby "sucked like a vacuum cleaner." She said that "if every baby sucked that way, most adoptive mothers would make milk!" And she was right, but she did not say that all such mothers will make a complete milk supply. If a mother has read stories of women who have done so, remind her that these mothers are the exception to the general rule. According to some reports, most adoptive mothers will make some milk, usually between twenty-five and seventy-five percent of a baby's total nutritional needs, prior to beginning solid foods.

Often, but not always, such mothers are able to reduce the amount of nonhuman milk they use in the tube-feeding device after their babies begin to eat solids. Should this occur, mother and baby will then be like all other breastfeeding mothers whose babies are also eating solids.

Remember: Whether a mother is relactating or inducing lactation, any amount of milk a mother's body makes confers protections the baby cannot obtain from nonhuman milks. However much milk the mother's body makes is proof that her baby is stimulating her body to make milk, and that her body is responding appropriately. Perhaps most important, nurturing a baby at the breast is making that baby a member of the family in a way that cannot be duplicated by any other means. Although a woman may not make as much milk as the birth-mother down the street who has not breastfed an adopted infant, or who never experienced an interruption of her breastfeeding experience, this does not make adoptive breastfeeding or relactation a lesser activity. Rather, induced lactation is simply different from breastfeeding a birth-child. And relactation is simply a variant on the original feeding plan. Each has its own unique qualities; each provides it own unique joys.

Kathleen G. Auerbach, Ph.D., I.B.C.L.C., is an adjunct professor at the School of Nursing, University of British Columbia, Vancouver, Canada, and a lactation consultant in private practice at the Parent Center in Ferndale, Washington. She is the co-author of *Breastfeeeding and Human Lactation* and four accompanying volumes, and editor-in-chief of *Current Issues in Clinical Lactation*, an annual volume. She was the first recipient of the International Lactation Consultant Association's Achievement Award in 1998 and the La Leche League International's 1999 Award of Excellence.

The use of medications in breastfeeding mothers is of concern to all professionals who work with these women, as well as to the women themselves. This chapter, with its thorough discussion of questions concerning medication and its listing of charts as well as its description of how medications work in breast milk, should be of value to everyone faced with these considerations.

Chapter 18
Medications and the Breastfeeding Mother

Thomas W. Hale, Ph.D.

Without doubt, one of the most divisive areas of clinical practice is the question arising from use of medications in breastfeeding mothers. Far too often, clinicians unaware of current data suggest that mothers who require medications should simply discontinue breastfeeding for variable periods of time. This suggestion is invariably discomforting to the mother, troublesome for the infant, and in many instances permanently it disrupts continued breastfeeding. This review aims to provide current information on the transfer of medications into breast milk during the perinatal or postpartum period, and the likely exposure of the infant to untoward effects.

DRUG TRANSMISSION INTO BREAST MILK

Drugs transfer into human milk largely as a function of their concentration in the maternal plasma compartment, their protein binding, lipid solubility, and molecular weight. Milk should be viewed as just another compartment where drugs enter, stay for a while, and then exit. Drugs enter the milk compartment and also, in almost all instances, exit via passive diffusion, or facilitated and/or active transport, which is largely determined by the equilibrium forces between the maternal plasma compartment and the milk compartment. As the concentration of drug in the maternal plasma increases, the drug is forced out of the plasma compartment into the milk compartment. Hence, a uniform standard is that as the plasma level rises, the milk level rises as well. Further, drugs that attain low levels in the maternal plasma compartment invariably produce minimal levels in milk as well.

In general, drugs with high protein bounding are also poorly transferred into milk, largely because, as they are sequestered in the maternal plasma compartment, they have difficulty exiting. In general, the more lipophilic a medication, the higher the level that is transferred to the milk compartment, but this again is largely dependent on the maternal plasma level. Drugs that have low molecular weights, such as lithium or ethanol, easily traverse the various tissue barriers and their rate and degree of entry into milk may be higher than other drugs. They may therefore attain higher levels than higher molecular weight drugs, although this is variable. Some chemicals may be actually pumped into milk via specialized cellular pumping systems. Iodine is a classic example and may have a milk:plasma ratio as high as 25. This is obviously a natural phenomena where the mother's alveolar epithelium is pumping extra iodine into milk to ensure proper neonatal thyroid function. In many ways, the secretory alveolar epithelium is similar to the blood-brain barrier, limiting the transfer of many drugs into milk, while permitting entry of others. As expected, drugs that enter the brain generally enter milk in higher concentrations as well, simply because most neuroactive drugs are highly lipophilic.

Another parameter commonly used is the milk:plasma ratio. As the ratio increases above one, it generally indicates that the medication is preferentially sequestered in milk at higher levels than in the maternal plasma. Although useful, the milk:plasma ratio is highly variable, depending on timing of the sample taken, the half-life of the medication, and the relationship of sampling to maternal peak. Further, it does not provide any information as to the absolute clinical dose of medication transferred to the infant. In instances where the maternal plasma level of the medication is exceedingly low, a correspondingly high milk:plasma ratio may still only suggest minimal transfer to the infant. Unfortunately, clinicians often interpret a high milk:plasma ratio to mean a high clinical dose to the infant, and this is not often true. Because many drugs with high milk:plasma ratios still produce subclinical doses to the infant via milk, the milk:plasma ratio may be a poor indicator of the actual dose delivered to the infant.

Oral bioavailability is a useful tool for determining the amount of a drug that is actually absorbed by the infant from the oral ingestion of milk. Although the GI tract of newborn infants is quite porous during the first few weeks of life, this changes with time and oral absorption kinetics of infants rapidly approach those of adults for many drugs. Further, while the liver of the newborn is quite immature at metabolizing drugs for at least several months, it appears very efficient at removing drugs from the plasma compartment and sequestering them in hepatic tissues. Poor oral absorption combined with prolonged storage in the liver is known to significantly reduce oral bioavailability of many medications in the neonate. Therefore, drugs that exhibit poor oral bioavailability often fail to produce clinical symptoms simply because they are not absorbed.

CALCULATING DOSAGE TO THE INFANT

Without doubt, the most useful determination of risk is the calculated dose to the infant. Using the peak milk levels published, and the weight of the infant, one can estimate the peak dose delivered via milk in twenty-four hours. Because it is often difficult to measure the daily milk intake, an average value of 150 milliliters per kilogram per day is often used to estimate daily infant milk. By multiplying the peak drug level in milk times daily milk intake as estimated from the body weight, one can estimate the peak daily dose delivered via milk. This is often a high estimate, but still quite useful.

Infant dose = peak concentration of drug in milk (in milliliters) X 150 milliliters X body weight (kg) X percent oral bioavailability/100.

However, this is only a poor approximation, as some infants may ingest as much as 230 milliliters of milk per kilogram, and the estimated maternal plasma drug level may be much lower, accounting for time periods when the maternal plasma levels reach a low, or trough, level.

EVALUATING INFANT SENSITIVITY TO MEDICATIONS

It should be quite obvious that certain infants are more sensitive to medications than others, including those passed through breast milk. Neonates, premature infants, those with poor hepatic and renal function, and those with specific pathologies such as severe apnea may be more sensitive to medications. Infants subject to apnea should not be exposed to depressant drugs, benzodiazepines, beta blockers, and sedating antihistamines without close monitoring. Neonates in the first month of life should not be exposed to sulfonamides, and other drugs with high protein-binding that might induce kernicterus. Ill and weakened infants should always be evaluated more closely prior to maternal drug use.

IDEAL KINETIC FACTORS

Choose drugs with shorter half-lives. Remember that the equilibrium forces which push drugs into milk are highest when the drug peaks in the maternal plasma compartment. Hence all drugs will be pushed into milk at higher levels when the mother's plasma level is maximum. Therefore, try not to breastfeed when the drug peaks in the mother's circulation. This is easier to do with medications that have short half-lives, as it is easier to wait several hours to breastfeed when the drug is at its lowest concentration; hence, only minimal amounts will transfer to the infant via the milk. Although not contraindicated, be more cautious of medications with long half-lives, or those who have long half-life active metabolites. Certain drugs (Prozac, Meperidine) when metabolized by the liver produce active metabolites with incredibly long half-lives, which can build up over time in the infant and produce side effects. But even with longer half-life medications (Phenobarbital, etc.), many of these can be safely used. Most fail to enter milk in high enough concentrations to produce clinical effects in the infant.

Medications with high protein-binding invariably have greater difficulty entering the milk compartment, simply because they are preferentially sequestered in the mother's plasma rather than entering milk. Drugs with high molecular weights have great difficulty penetrating through the alveolar epithelial cell and entering the milk compartment. Those with molecular weight above 800 to 1,200 daltons penetrate only poorly into human milk. Those with molecular weights above 2,000 to 4,000 are virtually excluded from milk. If possible, always choose drugs with the lowest oral bioavailability as this will invariably lower the total exposure of the infant; as the drug is either destroyed in the infant's gut, or sequestered in his liver, thus failing to attain plasma levels in the infant.

Ideal Drug Characteristics

Shorter half-life
High protein-binding
Poor oral bioavailability
High molecular weight
Low lipid solubility
Inability to enter the Central Nervous System

DRUGS WHICH DIRECTLY AFFECT MILK PRODUCTION

Some drugs may have profound effects on the production of breast milk, aside from their ability to enter milk. Some may potentially increase the production of milk, while others may profoundly suppress milk production. Early lactation is apparently highly sensitive to the level of circulating maternal prolactin. It is believed that those drugs which stimulate prolactin early on may increase the rate of breast milk production. Such drugs include metoclopramide, domperidone, and other dopamine antagonists. Drugs which stimulate dopamine levels in the brain may dramatically inhibit lactation, and include ergot alkaloids such as ergotamine, and cabergoline. Other drugs, such as estrogens, may produce local effects in the alveolar cell, and are well known for suppressing lactation if administered early postpartum.

SPECIFIC DRUG INFORMATION (SEE TABLE ONE)

Analgesics

The most commonly used analgesics in breastfeeding women are acetaminophen and ibuprofen. Both of these products are ideal, simply because the levels they attain in breast milk are largely subclinical and they are both cleared for pediatric use. Levels of ibuprofen transferred into milk following 400 milligram maternal doses are generally less than one milligram per liter of milk. Although some express concerns about the use of prostaglandin inhibitors due to their effect on closure of the ductus arteriosus in the neonate, we do not believe the dose transferred to the neonate is high enough to produce this effect. Acetaminophen levels in milk are reported to be only ten to fifteen milligrams per milliliter of milk. Long-acting nonsteroidals (NSAIDS) such as naproxen should be avoided, although they are not absolutely contraindicated.

Codeine and hydrocodone are often used for mild postpartum pain. Codeine is largely inactive while about ten percent is metabolized to morphine, which is the active analgesic. The amount of codeine transferred into milk is marginal, only about 140 micrograms per liter, although some reports of sedation and apnea have been reported with frequent 60-milligram doses. However, when the doses of codeine and hydrocodone were minimized, and administered after breastfeeding, few cases of neonatal sedation were reported. In many respects, morphine continues to be an ideal strong opiate for breastfeeding mothers in moderate to severe pain. Due to poor oral bioavailability (twenty-six percent), morphine produces only minimal sedation in breastfed infants. However, frequent and repeated exposure can lead to accumulation in the infant and should be avoided. The use of methadone both during pregnancy and postpartum is increasingly common primarily due to increased heroin abuse. While the AAP has approved the use of methadone in breastfeeding mothers who use twenty milligrams per day or less, this dose is seldom used anymore. Currently, doses approaching 80 to 120 milligrams per day are far more common. Fortunately, methadone has difficulty entering milk and, of the numerous studies with this analgesic, most seem to suggest the amount entering milk is minimal. Although one infant death has been attributed to this analgesic, other studies seem to suggest that even at higher doses the amount of methadone in milk is insufficient to prevent a neonatal abstinence syndrome (withdrawal).

Antihistamines and Decongestants

Antihistamines, sometimes in combination with decongestants, are often used by many breastfeeding women for treating cold symptoms or seasonal allergies. The older families of antihistamines, diphenhydramine (Benadryl), chlorpheniramine, and brompheniramine frequently produce significant sedation. Because sedation in a newborn infant may facilitate apnea, it is generally suggested that the nonsedating antihistamines are preferred. These include cetirizine (Zyrtec) and loratadine (Claritin). Most of the decongestants, pseudoephedrine, phenylephrine, and phenylpropanolamine are generally safe to use as long as the duration of exposure is not more than a few days. However, because many of these antihistamine/decongestant preparations are poorly effective for colds and flu symptoms, they may not prove beneficial enough to risk side effects in the infant, and therefore may not be justified. For treatment of chronic seasonal rhinitis, the use of long-acting, nonsedating antihistamines is sometimes recommended, but it is possible that due to their long half-lives, they could build up in infants over weeks of therapy. Another method, perhaps preferred, is to use the intranasal steroids. They are far more effective, and the risk to the breastfed infant is virtually nil, as most of these steroids have poor bioavailability and only small doses are applied topically to the nasal mucosa.

Antibiotics

Virtually all antibiotics are safe to use in breastfeeding mothers with perhaps the exception of the fluoroquinolone family and the sulfonamides at certain times. Penicillins, erythromycins, and cephalosporins enter milk only in trace levels and rarely produce allergies or changes in GI flora. Rashes, thrush, and diarrhea are the only likely consequences of exposure to these families of drugs. Third-generation cephalosporins are poorly bioavailable, and the only likely consequence of their use is diarrhea and overgrowth of *C. difficle*, which is uncommon. The fluoroquinolone family, which includes ciprofloxacin, ofloxacin, trovafloxacin, and others, are generally contraindicated in pediatric-age patients due to the reported arthropathy associated with their use. Although the levels transferred into human milk are probably too low to induce this pathology, they have been reported to induce overgrowth with *C. difficle* and one reported case of pseudomembranous colitis. However, a newer member, trovafloxacin (Trovan), transfers into milk in low levels (0.4% of maternal dose) and may be useful in breastfeeding mothers.

Sulfonamide drugs are seldom used during the last trimester of pregnancy and the first month postpartum, due to the potential for kernicterus. After the first month of life, sulfonamides are probably safe in most infants. Metronidazole, which is commonly used for trichomoniasis, giardiasis, and anaerobic infections, is controversial due to a theoretical risk of carcinogenicity. Reported levels in milk following maternal doses of 1,200 milligrams per day averaged fifteen micrograms per liter of milk, a level that is far less than the therapeutic dose of ten to twenty milligrams per kilogram commonly used in neonates and preterm infants. If required for trichonomiasis, a single two-gram dose following by interruption of breastfeeding for twenty-four hours is often suggested, although twelve hours may suffice. Metronidazole is so commonly used in pediatrics today, that the hysteria associated with its atheoretical carcinogenesis is usually dismissed. The tetracyclines can be briefly used in breastfeeding women. Many but not all are poorly absorbed while immersed in milk due to chelation with calcium salts. If the treatments are kept brief, then the amount transferred and the effect on skeletal growth and dental discoloration will be minimal to nil.

Antihypertensives

Typical antihypertensive families consist of the beta-receptor and calcium channel blockers, sympatholytics, ACE (angiotensin converting enzyme) inhibitors, and several others. Many of these agents have been thoroughly studied in breastfeeding mothers. Briefly, certain beta blockers such as acebutolol and atenolol have been associated with a higher incidence of hypotension and hypoglycemia in breastfed infants, and should be avoided. Propranolol and metoprolol are probably preferred, due to lower milk levels. But all infants exposed to the beta-blocker family should be closely monitored for apnea, weakness, and hypoglycemia. Of the calcium channel blockers, several members produce exceedingly low milk levels and should be preferred. These include verapamil, bepridil, nifedipine, and nimodipine. Hydralazine, which is commonly used in gestational hypertension, can be safely used in breastfeeding mothers, if the dose is moderate to low. The dose transferred in one liter of milk is approximately 0.17 milligrams, an amount too low to produce clinical effects in most infants. ACE inhibitors are more problematic. Due to extreme potency in neonates, they are universally contraindicated in the last trimester of pregnancy. Although the reported milk levels are low, the use of these agents in the early neonatal period is probably too risky. After one to two months' postpartum, captopril or enalapril can probably be used in the mother with due caution.

Antidepressants

With the introduction of the newer antidepressants, the number of patients receiving treatment for depression has risen extensively. Further, societal changes in the patients' own perception of antidepressant therapy have likewise changed

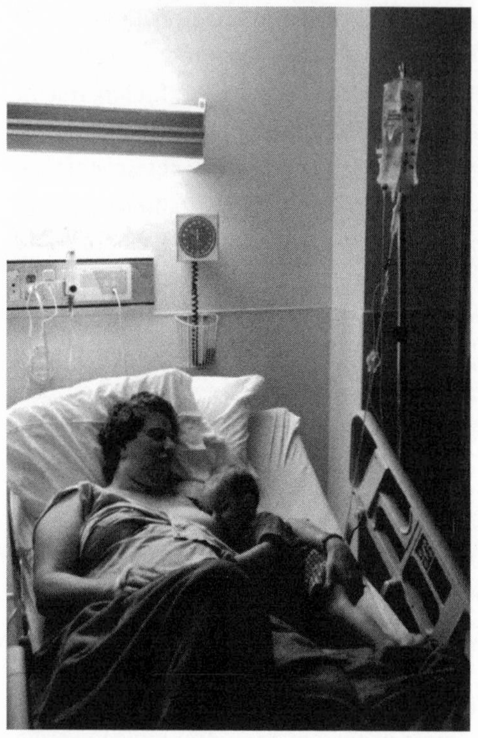

Mothers on medication or in hospital can often still breastfeed their child; it is safe to breastfeed with the great majority of medications. Among the exceptions to this are those cases in which the mother is being treated with various radioisotopes, certain anticancer drugs, and certain antibiotics.

so that now it is quite acceptable to seek and receive therapy for depression. Presently, about fifteen to twenty percent of postpartum women experience clinical depression, although about eighty percent will experience postpartum blues. In the past, the use of antidepressants has been controversial, with some reports of possible (but unpublished) neurobehavioral problems, while others, including the American Academy of Pediatrics, consider them acceptable in breastfeeding women. Recent evidence that depression may interfere with optimal parenting, and that infants of depressed women may suffer from developmental problems, has increased our urgency to treat this syndrome in certain breastfeeding women.

There are two major families of antidepressants that the clinician will encounter in breastfeeding mothers, plus a few other individual drugs. The tricyclic family, which includes amitriptyline, imipramine, desipramine and numerous others, is the oldest family of antidepressants. Of the more than forty published articles about various members of this family, almost invariably the amount of tricyclics transferred into human milk is quite low. However, this family is replete with untoward side effects in the mother, including constipation, sedation, dry mouth, blurred vision, and so on, so that patient compliance is often less than forty percent. In addition, the tricyclic family is horribly toxic in overdose, and most clinicians are reticent to dispense these drugs for patients who are already depressed and at risk for suicide. Thus far, neurobehavioral development of the breastfed infant exposed to tricyclic antidepressants (via milk) appears normal.

However, the most popular family of antidepressants is the serotonin reuptake inhibitors (SSRIs). This family consists of fluoxetine, sertraline, paroxetine, venlafaxine, and fluvoxamine. The largest selling member of this family is fluoxetine (Prozac) and is the subject of some concern. Fluoxetine is metabolized to an active, long half-life metabolite called norfluoxetine ($t^1/_2$= 300+ hours). This metabolite has been found in high levels in the plasma of several breastfed infants and has been correlated with a number of untoward effects such as colic, lengthy crying, increased vomiting, decreased sleep, watery stools, and coma. In addition, fluoxetine now has Federal Drug Administration clearance for use in pregnant women. This is of particular concern because infants born of mothers taking fluoxetine during pregnancy will be born with a full body burden of drug. In these cases, it is likely the small amount transferred in breast milk will continue to build to toxic levels. Fluoxetine should no longer be viewed as a preferred product in breastfeeding mothers with newborn infants.

The use of sertraline, on the other hand, has been reported in more than twenty breastfed infants, and appears to transfer poorly to the infant and with no side effects. Thus far plasma levels in most infants have been close to or below the limit of detection with no reports of untoward effects in the infant. At this time, sertraline is probably the SSRI of choice in breastfed infants. One case report of paroxetine use in a mother suggests that milk levels are exceedingly low and the amount transferred to the infant via milk would be minimal. In a study of three women using venlafaxine, milk levels were moderate providing 7.6% of the weight-adjusted maternal dose to the infant, but no side effects were noted in the infants.

The use of lithium in breastfeeding women has long been controversial. Lithium is a potent medication used in bipolar disorder to reduce manic symptoms, and is known to transfer into human milk in moderate levels. There have been several reports of side effects in breastfeeding infants, including cyanosis, T-wave abnormalities, and decreased muscle tone. Most studies generally suggest that plasma levels in breast fed infants are approximately thirty to forty percent of the maternal plasma level. From these studies it is apparent that lithium can permeate milk and is absorbed by the breastfed infant. If the infant continues to breastfeed, it is strongly suggested that he be closely monitored for serum lithium levels. Lithium does not reach steady-state levels for approximately ten days and clinicians may wish to wait at least this long prior to evaluating the infant's serum lithium level—sooner if symptoms occur. In addition, lithium is known to reduce thyroxine production, and periodic thyroid evaluation should be considered. One study suggests that lithium administration is not an absolute contraindication to breastfeeding, if the physician monitors the infant closely for plasma lithium.

Contraceptives

It has been well known for many years that estrogen-containing oral contraceptives may dramatically suppress lactation and infant growth. The estrogen component, if used early postpartum, is well known to significantly suppress lactation, leading to early supplementation and ultimately suppression of breastfeeding. The progestins in general do not suppress lactation in most women and medroxyprogesterone (Depo-Provera) has been used in many women with success, although some reports of milk suppression have been voiced. Because of this risk, it is often advisable to initiate contraception by using oral progestin-only mini pills for at least several months, followed by Depo-Provera at a later date in those women who are unaffected.

Corticosteroids

Steroid use should be categorized according to the method of administration: oral, inhaled, intranasal, or topical. The transfer of oral prednisone and prednisolone into human milk is generally quite low, and is dependent on the maternal dose. With extremely high maternal doses of 120 milligrams per day, breast milk levels varied from 54 to 627 micrograms per liter of milk, and only provide approximately forty-seven micrograms per day to the infant, an insignificant amount. The transfer of methylprednisolone into milk is equally minimal. In general, the absorption and bioavailability of topical, inhaled, and intranasal steroids is so low that these agents are unlikely to pose problems for a breastfed infant, simply because their oral bioavailability and the doses used are often minimal. Although the topical application of low-potency steroids directly to the nipple can be overdone, minimal and infrequent applications can be used without problems. Again, only low-potency steroid creams or ointments such as hydrocortisone or triamcinolone should be used.

Finally, steroids have potent and long-lasting sequelae in infants when misused, and the long-term exposure of breastfed infants to maternal steroids should be approached with a risk-versus-benefit assessment that includes length and duration of exposure, route of administration, and the overall maternal dose. The infant should be followed closely for appropriate growth and development parameters.

Herbal Medications

The use of herbal drugs is increasingly popular due to intense advertising and self-promotion. While they are frequently viewed as safer alternatives to conventional medications, this is not necessarily true, and particularly so for pregnant and breastfeeding mothers. Almost invariably, studies of herbal products are poorly done and their reported efficacy is often exaggerated. Herbals that contain anticholinergics, or more importantly the pyrrolizidine alkaloids, can be extremely dangerous and should be avoided. These include: chaparral, jin bu huan, germander, comfrey tea, mistletoe, skullcap, margosa oil, maté tea, pennyroyal oil, blue cohosh, and many others. One recent case of severe neonatal cardiomyopathy following therapy with blue cohosh in a pregnant woman has been reported and illustrates that herbal preparations are not innocuous. However, a number of other herbals with excellent safety profiles are known. One of particular interest is fenugreek. Commonly believed to be a galactagogue, no evidence of acute toxicity has been reported, nor has data been published that documents its galactagogue effect. The use of St John's Wort for treating depression is gaining in popularity. A significant body of literature exists with this product suggesting that it is relatively efficacious as an antidepressant and devoid of significant side effects. However, we do not know if it transfers into human milk, nor if it is safe in breastfeeding mothers. At this time, using herbal products while breastfeeding is, at best, risky, primarily due to our limited experience and knowledge of these interesting compounds in breastfeeding mothers. Herbal use in pregnant women should be avoided.

Vaccines

While most vaccines are administered to the infant, there are occasions when the breastfeeding mother may require vaccination, such as in women of childbearing age who are rubella negative, those who need influenza vaccines, or those who may be visiting foreign countries. It is known that living viruses, such as HIV, can be transferred to the infant via milk. While it is possible that even weakened (attenuated) viruses as used in vaccines can transfer to the infant, thus far no serious untoward effects have been reported. Most, if not all, vaccines are considered safe in breastfeeding mothers, and the Center for Disease Control (CDC) recommends that all vaccines can be safely used in breastfeeding mothers. In the past, there has been some concern about using live, attenuated virus vaccines as they were reported to induce mild symptoms of the disease. At least two studies have found rubella virus to be transferred via milk, although the presence of clinical symptoms was only modest. In general, the use of rubella virus vaccine in breastfeeding mothers of full-term, normal infants has not been associated with major untoward effects and is generally recommended if needed.

PUMPING AND DISCARDING MILK

It would extremely rare that a mother would need to pump and discard her milk, as most drugs maintain an equilibrium with the milk compartment and the maternal plasma. However, there are some occasions where complete cessation or short-term pumping and discarding the milk would be advisable. This is particularly important with various radioisotopes, certain anticancer drugs, and various antibiotics. For a complete description see Table 18-2.

CONCLUSION

In the last decade, it has become increasingly evident that breastfeeding provides enormous health benefits for human infants, with major reductions in pediatric disease, and enhanced neurobehavioral development. However, patients still encounter healthcare professionals that are hesitant to use medications in the breastfeeding mother because they are uncertain of side effects in the infant. So it has increasingly become the responsibility of the mother and other healthcare practitioners to educate the physician concerning this field. The best assessment of safety of a medication is first to review the published concentration of the drug in breast milk, and then to calculate the theoretical dose to the infant via milk. Using this technique, you can explain to the physician the dose the infant is likely to receive, and compare that to the mother's dose. For most medications, this information is readily available.

Breastfeeding just prior to administering the medication is often useful as well, for it invariably reduces the infant's exposure. Using shorter half-life drugs reduces the infant's exposure to higher maternal plasma levels and invariably reduces milk levels.

Finally, it is quite safe to breastfeed with the great majority of medications. The dose to the infant via breast milk generally averages far less than one percent of the maternal dose, which is often subclinical to the infant. In addition, one must always review the necessity of the medication itself. Some medications, such as the antihistamines, decongestants, antidiarrheal preparations, expectorants, and certain herbal drugs, are often poorly efficacious and may not be absolutely necessary; thus the mother should be advised to do without. By using a minimum of kinetic information and published milk levels, almost all mothers should be able to continue to breastfeed and use the necessary medications as prescribed.

Table 18.1. Partial List of Medications Contraindicated or of Concern:

Drug	**Effect on Lactation/Infant**
ACE inhibitors	High risk of hypotension in neonates
Acebutolol	Hypotension, hypoglycemia, apnea
Amphetamines	Anorexia, agitation; risk does not justify use
Anticancer agents	Possible immunosuppression/toxicity in neonate
Barbiturates	Monitor for infant sedation
Benzodiazepines	Chronic use may lead to infant sedation; dependence
Bromocriptine	Inhibits lactation; suppresses prolactin
Cabergoline	Inhibits lactation/prolactin
Cocaine	Infant cocaine intoxication
Corticosteroids	High dose, chronic use may reduce bone growth, etc.
Ergotamine	Inhibits lactation/prolactin
Estrogens	Suppress lactation early postpartum
Fluoroquinolones	Some may induce overgrowth of *C. difficle*; arthropathy
Fluoxetine	Colic, lengthy crying, increased vomiting, watery stools
Lithium thyroid function	Monitor maternal/infant plasma levels and
Lovastatin/others	Lowers cholesterol; risk does not justify use
Mebendazole	May inhibit early lactation
Methotrexate	Possible immunosuppression; neutropenia; GI accumulation
NSAIDS	Avoid long half-life NSAIDS; GI distress, diarrhea
Phenothiazines	May induce sedation, increase risk of apnea
Radioactive iodine	Accumulation in milk/breasts; thyroid toxicity/carcinoma
Tamoxifen	May inhibit early lactation

Table 18.2. Medications Where Pumping and Discarding of Milk Is Recommended

Medication	Recommended Period of Interrupted Breastfeeding
Iodine-131	Complete cessation for this child or infant
Iodine-123	24 hours for 10 mCi; 12 hours for 4 mCi
Iodine-125	Complete cessation for this child or infant
Tc-99m Pertechnetate	24 hours for 30 mCi; 12 hours for 12 mCi
Tc-99m RBC labeling	6 hours for 20 mCi
Tc-99m Sulphur Colloid	6 hours for 12 mCi
Tc-99m WBC	24 hours for 5 mCi; 12 hours for 2 mCi
Gallium-67	1 month for 4 mCi; 2 weeks for 1.3 mCi; 1 week for 0.2 mCi
Indium-111	1 week for 0.5 mCi
Thallium-201	24–48 hours following 111 mBq
Cisplatinin	3–7 days post infusion
Cocaine	24 hours
Metronidazole	12–24 hours following 2 gram dose only
Methotrexate	Complete cessation for this child
Cyclophosphamide	Complete cessation for this child
Doxorubicin	Complete cessation for this child
Phencyclidine (PCP)	Complete cessation for this child
Copper-64	50 hours

Thomas W. Hale, Ph.D., is Associate Professor of Pediatrics and Associate Professor of Pharmacology in the Division of Clinical Pharmacology at Texas Tech University School of Medicine and a leading authority on drug use and the breastfeeding woman. He is the author of *Medications and Mothers' Milk*, now in its ninth edition.

Breast cancer is a devastating diagnosis under any circumstances, but when it strikes at a young woman who hopes to have children and breastfeed them, it is particularly upsetting. This chapter thoroughly, realistically, and sympathetically discusses the possibilities and probabilities of breastfeeding after breast cancer.

Chapter 19
Breastfeeding After Breast Cancer

Pamela Berens, M.D., and
Edward Newton, M.D.

The devastating consequences of breast cancer seem to be highlighted when a mother with small children or a would-be mother suffers from breast cancer. The assault is directed at her core ethos, health, feminine definition, and primary supporting role in the family. Since one in nine women will be diagnosed with breast cancer, every woman has been exposed at some point to the anguish and suffering of a family member, friend, or acquaintance with the illness.

Women and their physicians are developing extensive diagnostic schemes to make early diagnosis of this common, threatening disease. Although a better use of epidemiology, better mammography, and the increased use of needle aspiration have reduced the frequency of breast biopsy, surgery remains one of the most common procedures. Naturally, many young breast cancer victims are asking about the effects of breast cancer therapy on a future pregnancy and lactation. This chapter will describe the consequences of breast cancer diagnosis and treatment on breastfeeding success.

PATHOPHYSIOLOGY

The relationship between breast surgery and subsequent breastfeeding is described by the degree that surgery causes distortion, obstruction, neuropraxis, and disruption of functional anatomy. Surgery and subsequent suture repair obstructs or distorts the collecting ducts of the breast. Each nipple is the outlet of fifteen to twenty collecting ducts that drain fifteen to twenty lobes. These ducts branch out in a radial fashion from the nipple and areola. In the sub-areolar area the ducts widen to create lactiferous sinuses where milk can be temporarily stored. As surgery is performed, these ducts and sinuses can be completely or partly obstructed by the surgical incision or suture repair. When the obstruction is complete the lactation ceases regardless of the degree of nipple stimulation. When the obstruction is partial, the milk output from the lobe(s) is proportionally decreased.

Clinically, partial obstruction presents localized engorgement and breast pain at the initiation of breastfeeding postpartum. If generalized engorgement is allowed to occur, the tissue edema obstructs the already compromised duct and a period of complete obstruction occurs. Within hours, back pressure reduces the alveolar gland's ability to produce milk and milk supply is reduced. As sufficient nursing reduces generalized engorgement, the duct may partially open. Nipple stimulation reactivates the glandular cells to increase milk production, tissue edema recurs, and milk production is reduced. The clinical pattern can describe a recurrent pattern of breast pain and soreness.

MASTITIS AND ABSCESSES

Mastitis and breast abscesses are a possible consequence of breast surgery. Stasis is a critical component of infection. Partially obstructed ducts fail to drain properly and a natural host defense is compromised. The rich media of retained milk is inoculated by the normal migration of microbes from the mother's skin or the infant's mouth. Subsequently, clinical mastitis and/or abscess develops. The stasis further compromises therapy of the infection by limiting adequate drainage and isolating the infected milk. Postinfectious scarring further compromises the lumen and recurrent mastitis is more common during the remainder of this lactational period and after subsequent pregnancies.

Nipple stimulation plays a necessary role in milk production. The frequency of nipple stimulation is proportional to the amount of prolactin secreted from the anterior pituitary. Absent or modified sensory input from the nipple/areola disrupts this critical link and milk production is proportionally reduced. Nipple stimulation also is critical to the "letdown" reflex. Nipple stimulation results in oxytocin release from the posterior pituitary. The oxytocin has a primary effect on the myoepithelial cells, which invest the alveolar glands of the breast. Under oxytocin stimulation, myoepithelial cells produce rhythmic contractions that force the stored milk through the ducts into the infant's mouth. As surgery often disrupts skin sensation (neuropraxis), the clinical result may be breastfeeding failure.

Oxytocin has a secondary role as a neurotransmitter, an important mediator of mother–infant bonding and love. When sensory nerves are cut during breast surgery, the release of oxytocin is reduced. The adverse outcomes as the result of a decrease in its concentration as the "hormone of love" are hard to study or define. Are they behavioral/society problems of childhood or adolescence?

SCARRING

The scarring from breast surgery, especially in the areolar area, may disrupt the functional anatomy of the nipple–areola complex. Normally, when the infant latches on to the breast, he or she molds the complex into a continuous teat using nipple and areola. A teat is formed by contraction of circular muscles under the skin of the nipple and areola. Nipple stimulation causes these muscles to contract and project the nipple outward. The lactiferous sinuses are pulled into the teat where the infant's tongue can strip the milk into its mouth. If the surgical scar limits the formation of the teat, the clinical outcome is poor latch-on with subsequent nipple trauma and pain.

BREAST BIOPSY

While screening mammography is routine in women over forty years old, monthly self-breast examination is recommended for all age groups. A distinct solid mass requires a histologic diagnosis. In pre-menopausal women the initial tool is a fine needle aspiration. A twenty- or twenty-two-gauge needle is inserted into the mass and aspirated. If fluid is obtained and the mass disappears, the patient is re-examined in three months. Greenish fluid usually indicates benign fibrocystic disease, whereas milk is most often found in pregnant or lactating woman. If the mass is solid, the mass is skewered several times under strong negative pressure. The goal is to obtain cells and/or small amounts of tissue for cytologic/histologic diagnosis. If no diagnosis can be made, a breast biopsy is necessary.

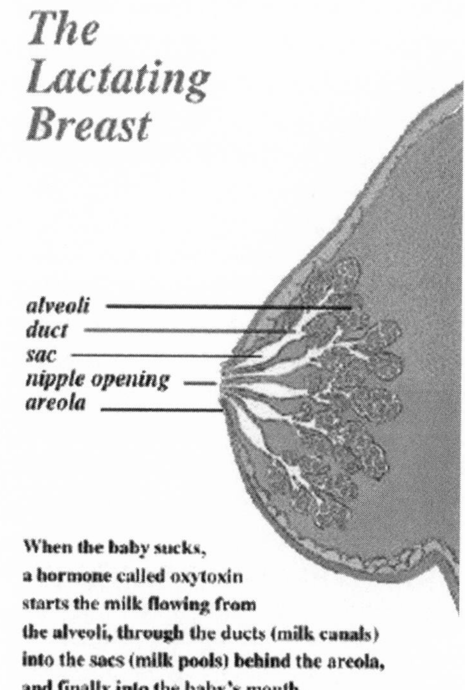

The Lactating Breast
alveoli
duct
sac
nipple opening
areola
When the baby sucks,
a hormone called oxytoxin
starts the milk flowing from
the alveoli, through the ducts (milk canals)
into the sacs (milk pools) behind the areola,
and finally into the baby's mouth.

Breast surgery always distorts the collecting ducts of the breasts so that when the nipples are stimulated, soreness and breast pain can be a problem.

While fine needle aspiration is an easy and potentially accurate outpatient screening procedure, the diagnosis rests on examination of tissue obtained by biopsy. Ellis and Cox prospectively evaluated 1,000 consecutive referrals for breast biopsy. Approximately 31% were normal, 22% were fibrocystic disease, 15% were simple cysts, 12% were carcinoma, 8% were fibroadenomas, and 2% were lipomas. The remainder was a mixed group. The age range for cancer was twenty-seven to eighty-three years with a mean of fifty-six years. The other diagnoses had mean ages well within the reproductive age group (mean ages, twenty-eight to forty-three years). All diagnoses were represented in postmenopausal women. Of these women twenty-one percent had previous benign breast disease.

CLASSIC SURGICAL TRAINING

If the mass is located within several centimeters of the areola, classic surgical training recommends a periareolar incision. As the ducts fan out in a radial fashion, the subcutaneous tissue is spread in a radial direction in order not to disrupt the ducts. After the removal of the mass, bleeding points are individually cauterized or ligated. Wide tissue-closing sutures are best avoided as the lactiferous ducts might be sutured or ligated.

In young women who anticipate having children and breastfeeding them, a periareolear incision is not appropriate. Periareolar skin incisions increase the likelihood of duct obstruction, tethering of the nipple, and neuropraxis. Obstruction, neuropraxis, and tethering of the teat are common consequences of periareolar and sub-areolar surgery. The degree of obstruction and limited teat formation by type of incision has not been measured. Periareolar surgery results in sensory loss in greater than forty percent of women.

Farina et al. studied the nerve supply to the nipple and areola. The lateral cutaneous branch of the fourth intercoastal nerve supplies the nipple complex from the four o'clock position on the left breast and the eight o'clock position on the right breast. By modifying their surgical approach in periareolar or trans-areola surgeries to a "ten to five o'clock" incision on the right nipple complex and a "seven to two o'clock" incision on the left, the authors were able to demonstrate fewer cases of neuropraxis.

BREASTFEEDING FAILURE

A prospective study of 319 primiparous women, among whom twenty-two had previous breast surgery, periaerolar skin incision (n = 10) was associated with a five-fold increase in breastfeeding failure. A retrospective study of women after surgical therapy for breast cancer demonstrated similar results. In young women who wish to breastfeed in the future, a skin incision in the periphery may be prudent. The cosmetic results of a radial skin incision or one parallel to the areolar edge are debated, but the incision of the subcutaneous tissue and its closure are similar to the periareolar incision.

A milk fistula is a rare complication after large core needle or sub-areola biopsy. In these cases, the biopsy enables the needle or incisional tract to become the fistula. This complication is most often seen in pregnant or lactating women. A milk fistula is more of an annoyance than a medical risk. The amount of leaking milk is usually small and often is controlled with a breast pad. The breastfeeding mother should not be dissuaded from breastfeeding based on the presence of a milk fistula. Most milk fistulas are self-limited over the course of several weeks.

LACTATION AFTER BREAST CANCER

One in nine women in the United States will get breast cancer (185,000 a year); most will be over the age of forty. Three percent of patients with breast cancer will be pregnant or lactating. Because of delay in diagnosis, a responsibility shared by patients and physicians, the prognosis is worse. The cumulative five-year survival is seventy-nine percent for age-matched non-pregnant and non-lactating women, and, fifty-five percent for pregnant or lactating women.

When stratified by node involvement, age-matched nonpregnant and nonlactating women had a cumulative five-year survival rate of ninety-three percent if there was no nodal spread, sixty-two percent with nodal spread. When the diagnosis is made during pregnancy or lactation, the cumulative five-year survival is eighty-five percent when there is no nodal involvement and thirty-seven percent when the nodes are involved at diagnosis. When breast cancer is diagnosed during pregnancy or lactation, approximately forty percent of breast cancer victims present with stage three or four disease as compared to age-matched women (thirty-six percent).

The diagnosis of breast cancer is devastating for the reproductive-aged woman. The thoughts of future pregnancy and lactation are placed on hold. The treatments for early breast cancer include mastectomy with prophylactic chemotherapy or lumpectomy with local radiation. During chemotherapy or during the period, when recurrence is likely to occur, pregnancy and lactation raise significant concerns. However, there is an increasing number of young women, three or more years after diagnosis and therapy, in whom pregnancy and lactation resurface as an issue.

There is no evidence that a history of breast cancer or its therapy affects the pregnancy. Likewise, pregnancy and lactation do not change the natural history of breast cancer. Therapeutic chemotherapy in women older than thirty years often results in premature ovarian failure. On the other hand, surgical and radiation therapy for breast cancer may complicate the success of breastfeeding.

There has been an increasing interest and use of conservative breast surgery and postoperative breast radiation therapy. Lumpectomy near or under the areola may compromise the lactiferous ducts such that breastfeeding from that breast may be impossible. Postoperative radiation directly affects the mammary glandular tissue within the radiation field. The number of functional alveolar units is markedly reduced, as is the maximum amount of breast milk that can be produced.

Breastfeeding after conservative breast surgery and radiation therapy is rare from the treated breast. Most of the literature consists of case reports of one to three patients. A survey of 2,582 members of the American Society of Therapeutic Radiology and Oncology[7] revealed fifty-three cases of pregnancy after conservative therapy from the eleven percent of members who responded.

It is apparent that women with a history of breast cancer avoid pregnancy and many avoid breastfeeding. Of those who make the positive choice, breastfeeding is most likely to be successful because the breast which did not receive therapy can supply plenty of breast milk. The survey revealed that eighteen percent were able to lactate from the treated breast and thirteen percent produced enough milk to adequately breastfeed from the treated side. In an interview survey of eleven patients with thirteen pregnancies after conservative treatment for early breast cancer, all patients reported breast asymmetry during pregnancy with the treated breast undergoing little or no enlargement. Two patients were not interviewed. Of the remaining women, lactation was suppressed after two pregnancies, not attempted in five, and attempted in four. Three of the four continued to breastfeed for four, sixteen, and twenty-eight weeks. All these patients reported reduced or no milk production from the treated breast. After four pregnancies (three patients), milk production was not observed from the treated breast where a periareolar incision had been performed.

Edward Newton, M.D., is Professor and Chairperson at East Carolina University, Brody School of Medicine. He received his medical degree and internship training at Loyola-Stritch School of Medicine in Maywood, Illinois, and completed his OB/GYN residency and fellowship training in Maternal-Fetal Medicine at Tufts University School of Medicine in Boston, Massachusetts. Dr. Newton has published three books, 83 abstracts, 59 articles, and contributed 29 chapters to other books.

Pamela Berens, M.D., is an Assistant Professor in the Department of Obstetrics, Gynecology and Reproductive Sciences at the University of Texas-Houston Medical School. She is on staff at Memorial Hermann Hospital and is the Medical Director at the Resident's OB/GYN Clinic. She is Board Certified in Obstetrics and Gynecology and a member of the Academy of Breast-Feeding Medicine.

Everyone knows that, under most circumstances, breastfeeding is best for both mother and baby. There are, however, rare contraindications for breastfeeding, of which HIV is probably the best known. In this clear, scholarly presentation, genuine and imagined reasons for not breastfeeding are thoroughly examined.

Chapter 20

When Not to Breastfeed: HIV and Other Infections

Ruth Lawrence, M.D.

Could there possibly be any contraindications to breastfeeding when we know that human milk is so right for the human infant? Could there be situations in which it is not in the best interest of the child to receive his mother's milk? While contraindications are often alluded to, there are actually very few real ones while the benefits of breastfeeding, as this book makes clear, are legion.

HIV POSITIVE AND AIDS

When considering possible contraindications to breastfeeding, therefore, decisions need to be made on an individual basis, weighing the tremendous benefit of breastfeeding against the risk of any possible contraindication. The most widely publicized contraindication to breastfeeding in the developed, industrialized world currently is immunodeficiency disease, or AIDS. The reason is that we don't know enough about the transmission of AIDS and we do know that the AIDS virus can be found in human milk.

Therefore, at present in the United States and other developed countries, it is recommended that women who are HIV positive do not breastfeed their infants. Current research on HIV has shown that the risk to the baby born to a mother with HIV can be reduced if she is provided with AZT medication prior to delivery and the infant is continued with this medication for the first few weeks of life. How this preventive program will ultimately affect the risk of breastfeeding is not yet known.

HTLV

The only other infectious disease that is a definite contraindication to breastfeeding is Human T-Cell Leukemia Virus Type I (HTLV). The incidence of human T-Cell Leukemia Virus Type I is increasing in parts of the world such as the West Indies, Africa, and southwestern Japan. There are only scattered cases in the United States.

Although the mother does not pass the disease to her unborn infant during pregnancy, it is felt that infected lymphocytes in her milk do contain the virus and could transmit the disease by breastfeeding.

OTHER INFECTIOUS DISEASES

There are a number of other infectious diseases that raise questions about the risks of breastfeeding. Top on this list is tuberculosis, which is increasing in frequency once again in developed countries due to the great migration from countries where it is very common. Breastfeeding is not contraindicated in women who have a positive skin test for tuberculosis but do not have any evidence of the disease. Oftentimes during pregnancy, the suspicion of active tuberculosis develops and efforts are made to establish the diagnosis before the mother delivers. Differentiation between a past tuberculosis infection and active disease is very important. If the disease is active, then it is urgent that the mother begin antituberculosis therapy immediately. This would include such medications as INH, rifampin, and pyrazinamide. The course of treatment lasts at least six months.

If a mother is on this therapy when she delivers her baby and she has no active chest lesions, it is safe for her to breastfeed her baby. Breastfeeding is not contraindicated if the disease is under treatment because the tubercle bacillus that causes tuberculosis does not appear in the breast milk. If the mother is considered contagious, the disease is transmitted by cough and sputum and a newborn baby must be separated from his mother in any case, whether the child is to receive her milk or be bottle-fed. The medications recommended are given to newborns and must be given to a baby whose mother has the disease. It is, therefore, safe to breastfeed while taking these medications as mentioned.

HEPATITIS

Hepatitis is another disease that has been of concern during pregnancy and breastfeeding. All hepatitis is not the same, however, and there are distinct differences in the management and prognosis of the different varieties. Hepatitis A is the acute illness, associated with fever, jaundice, and loss of appetite. It is usually acquired from contaminated food sources prepared by an individual with the disease. It is also appropriate when an outbreak is identified that all individuals who have been exposed to this case or this food handler receive gamma globulin. The local health department usually announces to the public this possible exposure. A newborn infant is rarely infected from his infected mother and it is safe to breastfeed as soon as the mother is well enough to do so.

Hepatitis B, however, can be present in a wide variety of stages of the disease from no symptoms at all to serious, or even fatal, hepatitis. Because we not only have hepatitis B immune globulin (HBIG), and there is now a vaccine to protect against hepatitis B, management recommendations have changed. When a mother with hepatitis B delivers, her baby is immediately given HBIG in the newborn nursery and the first dose of hepatitis vaccine is also administered before the infant is sent home. Breastfeeding is safe and actually recommended because of the tremendous benefits to the infant.

Hepatitis C is a separate entity, which has been identified with its own unique virus. Many adults with hepatitis C never recall being sick and are diagnosed because of a routine screening for insurance purposes, blood donation, or employment. As long as the mother is in good health, it is appropriate for her to breastfeed her baby even though she is hepatitis C positive. In the rare cases where a mother has serious hepatitis symptoms with jaundice and generalized illness, a decision about breastfeeding would have to be made based on the state of her disease.

HERPES SIMPLEX

Another infection of great concern to young women in the last few decades is herpes simplex virus. The recognition of herpes infections of the genital tract has alerted many people to the transmission of this virus and the possible risks to an infant. Newborn infants can acquire herpes during vaginal delivery if the mother has fresh lesions in her genital tract. On the other hand, if the mother is otherwise well and there are no lesions on her breasts, it is safe for her to breastfeed her healthy infant. Venereal warts, cytomegalovirus infections, and toxoplasmosis are not contraindications to breastfeeding.

ACUTE INFECTIOUS ILLNESS

A much more common situation is the mother who develops a respiratory infection or the common cold. Actually, her baby has been exposed to her germs before any significant symptoms develop. It is, therefore, better for the mother to continue to breastfeed her infant so that her baby will receive her antibodies through her breast milk and be protected against the disease and certainly its serious symptoms. In general, acute infections are not a contraindication to breastfeeding nor are they an indication to stop breastfeeding. It is better for the infant to receive the protective factors in the mother's milk than to be isolated from the mother and be deprived of this protection.

ACUTE MASTITIS

One specific disease is associated with breastfeeding and is of great concern to mothers. This disease, acute mastitis, an infection of the breast itself, is a victim of considerable misinformation about its management. Usually such an infection starts because a duct or a part of the breast becomes plugged and the blocked duct gets infected. The most important thing to remember about mastitis is to continue to breastfeed and to continue to breastfeed on the breast with the infection. While the mother should immediately notify her physician of the situation so that the doctor can prescribe appropriate antibiotics, it is also important to remember some simple guidelines for rapid recovery from mastitis.

One of the major reasons that women develop mastitis is that they are fatigued or rundown. A new mother's resistance is often lowered and she develops a local infection in her breast, runs a fever, and feels as if she has the flu. Part of the treatment is adequate rest. The mother must recognize that she cannot do all of her housework and all of the things she was trying to do and should concentrate on getting adequate rest and recuperating. She should take the antibiotics prescribed for her faithfully for the full length of time because of the possibility of recurrence of the infection or the development of chronic mastitis when antibiotics are taken for an insufficient length of time.

MEDICATIONS AND PRESCRIPTION DRUGS

Much concern and anxiety has been expressed regarding the question of medications taken by lactating women and the risk of these medications to the suckling infant. In truth, however, very few drugs are actually contraindicated during breastfeeding. Each situation should be evaluated on a case-by-case basis by the woman's physician. When prescribing for a woman in the childbearing years, it's important for the physician to inquire about pregnancy and lactation and conversely it's important for women to remind their doctors when they are either pregnant or lactating.

The American Academy of Pediatrics (AAP) has prepared a brief list of common medications that might be taken by a lactating woman. The AAP Committee on Drugs has divided medications into categories according to their risk to a breastfed baby. The first list includes drugs that are not recommended during breastfeeding. This list is short and includes medications that are uncommonly used and are particularly restricted to patients who are being immunosuppressed because of various cancers or transplant of major organs. A second table includes a list of radioactive compounds that are used for diagnostic purposes with only one dose of radioactive material. The recommendation is that breastfeeding should be temporarily discontinued, the milk pumped and discarded, until the radioactive material has cleared the mother's system. The information is readily available on the length of time that a mother should pump and discard her milk, depending on what radioactive material she has been given. The recommendations vary from twelve hours to several weeks. When it is necessary for a women to have such a compound while lactating, her physician should tell her how long she needs to pump and discard her milk.

STREET DRUGS AND TOBACCO

A third group of drugs considered contraindicated during breastfeeding by the AAP are so-called street drugs. The list is short and includes amphetamines, cocaine, heroin, marijuana, and phencyclidine. Caution is recommended for cigarette smoking. Although it is better for a mother not to smoke while pregnant or lactating, it is well documented that if a mother cannot abandon her habit, it still is better for the infant to be breastfed by a smoking mother than bottle-fed. Sudden Infant Death Syndrome (SIDS) occurs more commonly among infants whose mother or parents smoke than infants who live in households without any smokers. But when an infant is breastfed, it mitigates this risk. Infants who are breastfed also have fewer respiratory illnesses when their parents smoke than do bottle-fed infants of smoking parents.

ALCOHOL

Alcohol (ethynol) presents another series of questions. In many countries of the world alcoholic beverages such as wine and beer are consumed daily with meals, where breastfeeding is universal. On the other hand, there is concern about the chronic use of hard liquor while breastfeeding. It is advised by the Subcommittee on Lactation of the Institute of Medicine that a lactating woman limit her intake to no more than one half-gram of alcohol per kilogram of maternal body weight per day. These figures translate into a sixty-kilogram (132 lb) woman taking one half-gram of alcohol per kilogram per body weight or two to two-and-a-half ounces of hard liquor, eight ounces of table wine, or two cans of beer per day. It is recommended that lactating mothers stay within these limits.

DRUGS FOR COMMON ILLNESSES

Most drugs necessary to treat the common illnesses of women in the childbearing years are safe during lactation. Most importantly aspirin, acetaminophen, and ibuprofen—drugs commonly used for fever, generalized aches and pains, and upper respiratory infections—are safe during lactation. Cold preparations, which are intended to dry secretions, should not be taken during lactation because of their tendency to also decrease the milk supply. Antibiotics, on the other hand, are generally safe during lactation. There are only a few antibiotics that are not recommended for infants and children and those should be avoided during lactation.

Should a mother need a particular prescription medication she should discuss the fact she is breastfeeding with her physician. If her physician requires further information regarding medications he wishes to prescribe, he can contact the Breastfeeding and Human Lactation Study Center in Rochester, NY, at (716) 275-0088. This is a special service for physicians to provide information about special issues of breastfeeding and human lactation. The physician will want to take into consideration the magnitude of the risk of the drug compared to the tremendous benefit of being breastfed. This decision is made on a case-by-case basis and a physician should consider this for each individual mother and baby dyad.

HERBS AND HERBAL PRODUCTS

As we blend more cultures and more traditions from around the world, the topic of herbs and herbal teas has become a frequent topic for discussion. Much of the traditional and current use of herbs surrounds pregnancy, childbirth, and lactation. While many herbal teas contain innocuous flavors, others contain pharmacologically active components that form the basis for folk medicine treatments. A number of natural herbs contain real medications. A well-known one is digitalis, the traditional heart medication which can be found in the well-known American flower the foxglove. Other herbs contain naturally occurring coumarins, which are anticoagulants, and their excessive use can lead to bruising and hemorrhage. Comfrey leaves have been a favorite of traditional midwifery but have been banned in Canada and other countries because the use of comfrey has been associated with a serious liver disease and veno-occlusive disease.

The herb echinacea, which is widely touted as a preventive for colds and respiratory illness, is relatively innocuous if taken in modest amounts for short intervals. It may be safer during lactation than some of the over-the-counter cold preparations. Fenugreek is another popular herb; it has been credited with increasing milk supply although there are no good scientific studies to confirm this. In modest amounts, fenugreek is considered safe during lactation. St. John's Wort has achieved great recognition recently because it has been used, particularly in Germany, as an antidepressant. It does have significant pharmacologic properties and has been shown in some studies in Europe to be effective against postpartum depression. When taken cautiously under the care of a physician, it is considered as safe as some of the anti-depressant prescription medications. Its use should be discussed with a physician so that the proper diagnosis is made and some control over dosage is provided. No herbs should be taken casually.

BABIES WHO SHOULD NOT BREASTFEED

Mother's milk and breastfeeding provide the ideal nutrition and opportunity to receive special immune protection; however, there is one newborn disease that contraindicates breastfeeding and that is galactosemia. This disease involves the absence of the enzyme that is important in the digestion and utilization of lactose. Lactose is milk sugar and all mammalian milks contain some lactose. Infants who do not have this enzyme are unable to metabolize lactose, and this causes serious problems. Galactosemia is a very different disease from lactose intolerance. Lactose intolerance does not occur in newborns or in infancy. It is related to the gradual disappearance of another enzyme in the intestinal tract.

Controversy Over Call For Aids Moms To Breastfeed Babies

By Fanyana Mabuza

Mbabane, Swaziland September 18, 2000 (African Eye News Service (Nelspruit))—In a posture reminiscent of President Thabo Mbeki's controversial stance on HIV/Aids, Swaziland's health minister has urged mothers to breastfeed —even if they are HIV-positive.

"It is worrying to hear about the possible transmission of the Aids virus through breastfeeding. So much has been achieved in teaching the gospel of breastfeeding to Swazi mothers," health minister, Dr Phetsile Dlamini, said. "Breastfeeding is a right that should be enjoyed by every child without the threat of poverty, and all social ills including the advent of HIV/Aids," she added.

Dlamini was speaking at the close of the 5th International Baby Food Action Network (IBFAN) conference, held in Ezulwini, outside the capital city of Mbabane this week. Earlier, participants at the conference reinforced the position that breastfeeding could lead to mother-to-child transmission of HIV, the virus that causes Aids.

But the health minister's position has been backed by the Swaziland Infant Nutrition Action Network (SINAN). While conceding that it raised the possibly of HIV-transmission to infants, the organisation said the benefits of breastfeeding outweighed the dangers.

"There is a 14 percent chance of mothers passing HIV to their children through breastfeeding. However, the possibility of children dying of poor nutrition because of a lack of breastfeeding is higher," SINAN administrator Marie Hallisay said in an interview.

"Most mothers can not afford substitute foods," she added.

An estimated 22 percent of Swaziland's 980 000 people are believed to be HIV-positive.

Research is still being conducted to determine when it is not beneficial for HIV positive mothers to breastfeed their babies. Preliminary findings suggest that treatment with AZT alters the benefits of breastfeeding.

Individuals with lactose intolerance usually were able to drink milk as children but later gradually developed gastrointestinal symptoms including gas and diarrhea when exposed to large amounts of lactose. This intolerance can sometimes be improved by consuming dairy products that contain the enzyme lactase.

Galactosemia and lactose intolerance are two different diseases. Galactosemia is a contraindication for breastfeeding in most cases, unless the infant has a very mild deficiency of this blood enzyme. Other disorders involving amino acid enzyme deficiencies such as phenylketonuria (PKU) are managed differently depending on the disease and the individual child. In the case of PKU disease, the child is breastfed part of the time and receives a small amount of phenylalanine free milk or Phenylac.

SUMMARY

Contraindications to breastfeeding are extremely rare. They include active immunodeficiency disease (HIV) in the mother or HTLV in the mother. There is a short list of drugs that are contraindicated during lactation and a rare metabolic disease in the infant that could be a problem. In general, as the Institute of Medicine has stated, all infants in the United States under ordinary circumstances should be breastfed.

Ruth Lawrence, M.D., is the author of *Breastfeeding: A Guide for the Medical Profession*, now in its 4th edition. She is Professor of Pediatrics, Obstetrics and Gynecology at the University of Rochester School of Medicine in Rochester, New York. She is frequently asked to lecture based on her trailblazing paper "A Review of the Medical Benefits and Contraindications to Breastfeeding in the United States."

Although United States breastfeeding goals of 75% initiation and 50% continuation of any breastfeeding at six months are far from being realized, there is a potential of at least $3 billion for the health system and an additional $2 billion in household savings if these goals are reached.

Chapter 21

Cost Benefit of Breastfeeding in the United States

Is Supporting Exclusive Breastfeeding Worth the Costs?

Miriam H. Labbok, M.D., M.P.H.

Breastfeeding has been one of the Health Goals for the Nation since 1980, when the Surgeon General called for increases in the incidence and the duration of breastfeeding by 1990. Nonetheless, there was a net decline in breastfeeding initiation between 1980 and 1990. The goal was increased for the year 2000, planning for 75% initiation of breastfeeding and 50% continuation at 5–6 months. By 1993, the initiation had risen, returning to the level in 1980, while continuation of breastfeeding to 5–6 months rose from the low 20s to about 30.8% Today, we are seeing real increases in the segments of the population that were least likely to do breastfeeding in 1990. While the rate of breastfeeding among whites has increased by about 17% over the last 10 years (from high 50s to 67.9%), the rates among Hispanics has increased by nearly 40% (from the high 40s to 66.2%) and blacks have increased breastfeeding introduction by 100% (from the low 20s to 44.9%) (see Fig. 1). This underscores the responsiveness of breastfeeding behaviors to appropriate support and counseling.

The goals for breastfeeding in the U.S. have changed little in the last 20 years. Currently, the goals are 75% initiation and 50% continuation of any breastfeeding at six months, and are far from being reached. The findings that demonstrate the importance of exclusive breastfeeding have not yet been included in the goals. This is due, at least in part, to the fact that research on the impact of breastfeeding in the United States has rarely included sufficient definition of the breastfeeding pattern to allow differentiation in this regard. Where study findings differ, it is not infrequently due to insufficient controls or variable definitions of breastfeeding.

WHAT ARE THE COSTS?

In order to succeed in exclusive breastfeeding, a mother needs to be with her child and to receive whatever support is necessary to ensure that she has the

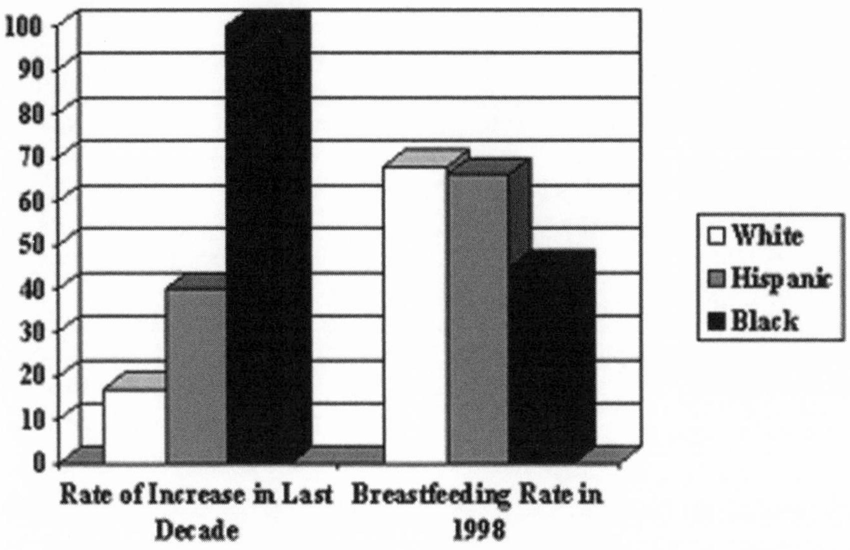

Figure 1: Rate of Increase in Initiating Breastfeeding in the Last Decade and Recent Rates of Initiation, in Percent by Group. Derived from Child Health USA 2000, USDHHS, HRSA/MCHB, p. 18.

skills necessary to achieve her intentions. Therefore, to support exclusive breastfeeding (defined as on demand, no other food or liquid, directly from the breast), women need to be with their child full-time, and to be able to access and afford the services of qualified professionals if needed. Both of these can be major issues separating intentions from success. While a few workplaces endorse bringing the child to work, most are still hesitant. Until this becomes the norm, each mother will have to find the time away from work to be with her child. Exclusive breastmilk feeding (defined as no other food or liquid except the mother's milk, direct or stored) is a currently accepted approach; however, for the immunological components of the milk to be in synch with the needs of the infant, the mother and child must be exposed to the same pathogens, and therefore, preferably, should be together, especially in the early weeks when supply is being established. And there may be a considerable personal and financial cost of staying home even for 12 weeks.

Another major issue for breastfeeding success in the United States, where the skills in the techniques of breastfeeding were nearly lost in the 1960s and 70s, is the limited availability of skilled professional support and the limited reimbursement available from standard insurers. Without reimbursement, there is less incentive for the professional to develop the skills and offer the needed services.

Third-party payment support for breastfeeding remains a rarity; breastfeeding support seems to decline under capitation schemes that have become very popular. In order to complement voluntary support with a health team as needed, the costs of training and reimbursement must be considered.

WHAT ARE THE BENEFITS?

The issue of breastfeeding is complex. The World Health Assembly of World Health Organization (WHO) and the Blueprint for Action on Breastfeeding of the Surgeon General of the United States both recommend exclusive breastfeeding for about six months. Both also recommend continuing breastfeeding with supplement for one or two years or more. The United States Agency for International Development (USAID) supports this pattern of breastfeeding, as well as the Lactational Amenorrhea Method for family planning, in order to impact both on maternal/child health and on birth spacing. UNICEF, with its support for Baby-Friendly Hospital Initiative, is increasing worldwide attention to the benefits of breastfeeding for every child.

One recent study in Russia reconfirmed both the effectiveness of the BFHI approach and the positive health outcomes that accrue. These benefits include decreased infectious disease, including respiratory, gastro-intestinal and inner ear, improved vision and other developmental parameters, improved dental health and excellent nutrition. Chronic diseases, including diabetes and other gastrointestinal syndromes as well as childhood cancers and possibly autoimmune disease, are reduced. SIDS, the major cause of postneonatal infant mortality, can be significantly reduced. Recent studies have indicated that breastfeeding is associated with increased intelligence and improved behavior. Not as well known are the benefits for the mother, including improved postpartum recovery, decreased ovarian cancers and probable decreases in osteoporosis and breast cancer. Overall, the evidence is clear that breastfeeding conveys both immediate and long-term positive health effects for both the child and the mother.

WHAT IS COST/BENEFIT ANALYSIS?

Given that breastfeeding is an important behavior for healthy outcomes for both mother and child, and given that there are certain costs involved in its support, how can we assess that the cost savings that occur if breastfeeding increases is worth the costs of the effort to provide the necessary support to achieve improved breastfeeding? Fiscally, this may be examined in a cost-benefit analysis (CBA). To develop the data on savings that would accrue and the costs of support, it is necessary to define and model the costs and savings, use whatever information is available to test the models, feed the estimates into a CBA formula and further refine it as more information becomes available.

Models to estimate costs and benefits were developed based on standard cost analysis techniques, assessing costs and benefits with a variety of assumptions. The results of the models are then incorporated into a standard cost benefit equation that has been modified to apply to this issue.

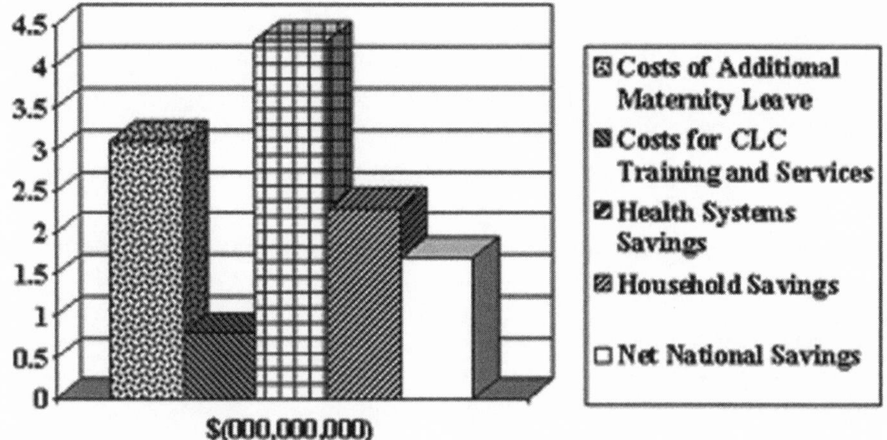

Figure 2: Expenses and Savings Associated with Supporting 12 Weeks Exclusive Breastfeeding in the USA.

WHAT ASSUMPTIONS WERE USED?

Terms used in this study are based on a widely accepted schema for definition of breastfeeding. Exclusive breastfeeding means that no other liquid, solid or feeding apparatus was used to feed the child. Exclusive breast-milk feeding is when breast milk is the only liquid or solid consumed by the infant. Since many of the studies used to estimate impact did not make this differentiation, some of the relative risks may be conservative.

For all calculations it is assumed that no infant is exclusively breastfed for 12 weeks in the U.S. today. Actually the figure may be about 3–4% at one month, dropping rapidly thereafter; however, this is not considered herein due to the low level and dearth of accurate data on exclusive breastfeeding patterns in this country.

There are limitations to these analyses. First, the inattention to this issue in the past and the funding of interest groups, such as formula companies, to collect the national data on breastfeeding, leaves us today with a limited profile of breastfeeding behaviors. Second, national costs of treating specific illnesses in infancy are not available, and for the most part, when they are retrievable, calculations are made using average charges rather than actual costs. And, third, it is difficult to apply a dollar amount to effects such as improved rates of survival or lives saved. Nonetheless, sufficient data are available to estimate several of these parameters and to calculate estimated costs.

With demonstration of the potential impact of breastfeeding as a health intervention, policy-makers may choose to modify the parameters of U.S. data collection on breastfeeding and related health sequelae in the future. As better data become available, all of these calculations may be improved.

WHAT WERE THE COST AND BENEFITS? AND WHAT IS THE RESULT OF A CBA?

There are several costs in supporting breastfeeding in the United States today.

1. The first area of costs is that engendered by the need to stay in physical proximity to one's child, often necessitating leave from work. The total U.S. estimated cost of sufficient additional leave to permit 12 weeks for mother and child to be together for exclusive breastfeeding is estimated at $3.1 billion.
2. Second, and equally important, are the health system costs of creating and maintaining the skilled support needed to reestablish a breastfeeding norm and to prevent and overcome obstacles to successful breastfeeding. This is estimated as $763 million.

Benefits accrue to the health system in terms of

1. reduced health costs of treating excess illnesses associated with non-breastfeeding, and
2. reduced outlay by the household for related commodities.

These are estimated in a variety of ways and averaged as about $4.2 billion and $2.331 billion, respectively.

Using the model described in the appendix, one can subtract the dollar amount of the benefits from the dollar amount of the costs for a net gain or loss. The combined cost of supporting the mother's time and the breastfeeding is $3.09 billion plus $0.763 billion = $3.853 billion. The savings, using an average of the models provided, are over $4 billion. In addition, savings at the household level, even when extra food for the mother is taken into account, are more than $2 billion. Therefore the cost/benefit calculation, including maternal support and disease reduction, yields a net excess of over $0.5–2.7 billion dollars. When set up as a cost/benefit ratio, we find a ratio of about 0.57 to 0.9, depending on which costs and benefits you include. To the country as a whole, this means a potential savings of $1.11 to $1.73 for every dollar invested in a combined effort of breastfeeding support and maternity leave. *See fig. 3.*

For insurance companies, which, in all likelihood, would not cover maternity leave, the costs would be the Lactation Consultant (LC) support only. Assuming that there would be need for additional support if maternity leave cannot be guaranteed, the costs might be increased by $200 per birth, or a total of $1.432 billion for LC training and services. If this is sufficient to persuade women to take the time to breastfeed for 12 weeks on their own, the savings for the healthcare system would remain at about $4.2 billion, for a cost savings to the public and private insurers and HMOs nationwide of about $2.5–3 billion. Stated as a cost/benefit ratio of 0.43, the insurance and other third-party approaches would save $1.55 cents for every dollar spent.

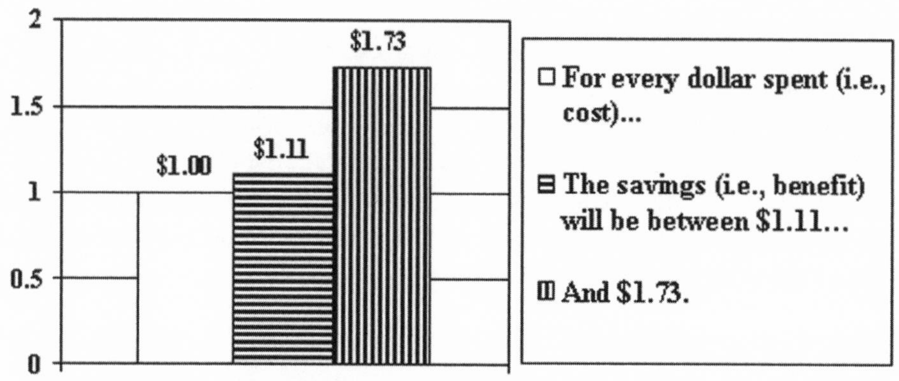

Figure 3: Cost-Benefit Analysis

HOW DOES THIS COMPARE TO OTHER FINDINGS?

While this analysis was originally completed and presented in 1993, there have been few major advances in fiscal support by third-party or HMO providers for breastfeeding per se. Analyses continue to show the vast cost saving that would accrue if infants were breastfed. A recent analysis by Weimer, which looked at the Health for the Nation recommendations rather than at exclusive breastfeeding, found similar results. While this paper includes costs of some infant infections, diabetes, neoplasia and chronic GI disease, the Weimer study only includes otitis media, gastroenteritis and NEC, and still finds, "A minimum of $3.6 billion would be saved if breastfeeding were increased from current levels (64 percent in-hospital, 29 percent at 6 months) to those recommended by the U.S. Surgeon General (75 and 50 percent). The study goes on to state that this is an underestimate due to the small selection of illnesses. Indeed, if the chronic illnesses from the model in this paper were added, the gross total would surpass $7 billion.

Why, then, with several powerful analyses available, do the cost savings of breastfeeding, and the excess costs of non-breastfeeding, remain so UN-noticed by insurer and health policy makers? Jane Heinig addressed this issue in her excellent editorial "Breastfeeding and the Bottom Line: Why Are Cost Savings of Breastfeeding Such a Hard Sell?" She explains that policy-makers can easily dismiss the hypothetical approach, when one assumes that rates and costs apply widely. However, in this analysis, the data are based on population findings for the most part, and therefore much of the potential confounding is internally controlled. Nonetheless, there is much room for discussion of every figure used.

This paper attempts to take the discussion one step further: to assess both the benefits and the costs of supporting breastfeeding nationwide. There are real and measurable costs in any behavior choice. There are also real and unmeasurable costs, such as day-to-day emotions, or, much worse, the impact on a family of the loss of a child. In this paper, only the measurable costs have been considered. Nonetheless, the net savings and the benefits per unit cost, with even these conservative estimates, are huge.

SUMMARY: ARE WE ABLE TO ACT?

Breastfeeding is recognized as saving millions of lives each year worldwide, but coverage for its support and maintenance are not included in most healthcare plans. A major issue for those who provide support for breastfeeding is reimbursement for that service. Few third-party or HMOs currently cover these costs. To examine this issue, it is necessary to see what information is available, develop the defense, and further refine the approach as more information becomes available. Three models were used to examine the potential cost savings of as little as 12 weeks of breastfeeding in the United States, two based on health systems savings due to decreased disease and one based on household savings. The models reveal potential cost savings of over $4 billion for the health system and an additional $2 billion or more in household savings. Estimated costs of the support necessary to enable women to succeed in their choice to breastfeed are also discussed, with a range of $632 million to $20 billion, but a reasonable approach at about $3.2 billion.

The conclusion is that increased support for breastfeeding would have a positive cost-benefit outcome, with a national net cost savings of at least $0.5–2.7 billion annually. It is important to consider the implication of these results in terms of institutionalization of support (e.g., third party payment, hospitals services, community), national legislation and regulation and the need for better data.

In sum, breastfeeding is a vital component of our health system, and should be supported and acknowledged for its contribution to the health of our nation. And putting dollars behind this will only serve to result in significant cost savings over time. Can we think in terms of lifetime planning in our health systems? Can we escape the business school mentality of 2–5 year profit expectation? The question for today, then, is not whether breastfeeding would result in cost savings, better health and a better future, but whether we, as a nation, can truly address and act upon a social/health issue that demands up-front investment for a potential savings, and for a healthier future

ACKNOWLEDGMENTS:

This paper was presented, in part, at previous meetings including: The APHA annual meeting, San Francisco, October 25, 1993, and PREVENTION 93, April 18, 1993, St. Louis, Mo.; the ILCA meeting in Scottsdale, 1995; a BSC in Nashville, 1997; and others. Parts of the paper were published as Labbok M. *Cost Effectiveness of Breastfeeding in the United States.* (*ABM News and Views*,1995, 1(1):6). This paper reflects the opinions of the author and does not necessarily reflect the viewpoints of Georgetown Medical Center or of the United States Agency for International Development. Aspects of this analysis will be submitted for publication in a refereed journal.

Dr. Miriam H. Labbok, M.D., M.P.H., currently serves as Medical Officer and Chief, Nutrition and Maternal/Infant Health Division, at the United States Agency for International Development, and is Adjunct Associate Professor at Johns Hopkins and Tulane Schools of Public Health. Previously she served as Assistant Professor at the Johns Hopkins School of Hygiene and Public Health and Associate Professor at Georgetown University Medical Center.

Appendices

APPENDIX 1: ASSUMPTIONS AND CALCULATIONS OF COSTS AND BENEFITS

Miriam H. Labbok, M.D., M.P.H.

COST OF MATERNITY LEAVE (CMT)

Cost of Maternity Leave (CMT) = $(T \times C_T \times W)$

Where T = number of units of time for leave

C_T = Cost per unit of time

W = Number of women potentially in the workforce

The U.S. per capita income at the time of this analysis was approximately $22,560, just slightly lower than Sweden's at $25,490. Costs are calculated using the Swedish maternity leave approach of 90% of income for the first year, and $8 per day for longer periods, as well as U.S. minimum wage income of about $5.15 per hour, or $10,300 for 50 forty-hour weeks. There are about 150 million women in the workplace, or about 40% of the labor force, but this might well increase if maternity leave were supported. There are well under 4 million births per year, and if we assume that just under $^2/_3$ of these are to women in the workforce, that yields an estimate of about 2.5 million working women facing maternity leave decisions annually.

The cost of supporting 12 weeks or 90 days of leave in the U.S. is calculated at three levels, assuming a significant increase in women in the workforce if paid maternity leave were established:

Model CMT_1: Where T is 0.25 year, C_T is $22,5600, and W is 3 million, CMT_1 = $16.92 billion.

Model CMT_2: Where T is 60 days, C_T is $8, and W is 3 million, CMT_2 = $1.44 billion.

A more realistic assumption might be the attainment of six weeks additional leave at minimum wage for women currently employed,

Model CMT_3: Where T is 0.12 years, C_T is $10,300, and W is 2.5 million,
CMT_3 = $3.1 billion.

COST OF "LACTATION CONSULTANT" SUPPORT

Since it may be assumed that there are not a sufficient number of trained physicians, nurses or practicing lactation consultants, the cost of providing breastfeeding support must include:

1. the cost of training the new skilled cadre, and,

2. the cost of the services provided.

It is recognized that this will yield a high estimate of the cost in this category, since the costs of training are not usually included.

Cost of Support (CS) = (D x T_D) + (C_D x P)

where D = the number of full-time equivalent designated lactation consultants needed
T_D = Cost of training a designated LC or M.D.
C_D = Average cost of LC/M.D. breastfeeding support
P = Population at risk, or number of live births

If we assume there is a need for one full-time equivalent lactation support person, whether certified lactation consultant, trained nurse or trained physician, for every 1,000 births, or about 4,000 for the nation. Currently there are more than 3,000 Certified Lactation Consultants and a growing number of trained physicians and nurses. Therefore, the main costs include some additional training (1,000 CLCs and 1,000 physicians for 150 hours at $10 per hour or $3.0 million) plus a high average estimate of the cost per infant for all infants at about $200, or $760 million.

Where D is 2,000, T_D is $1,500, C_D is $200, and P is 3.8 million, CS = $0.763 billion

Benefits of breastfeeding (savings) are the estimated savings related to breastfeeding. The benefits are calculated based on three models: Disease-based Model, Health Expenditure Model, and Household Expense Model.

Disease-based model

Benefit (B_D) = _ k_x (I_x x P_x x R_x x C_x)

where k_x = constant for number of years of effect of disease x
I = Incidence of disease x
P = Population at risk of x, or number of live births

R = Reduction in rate of x associated with breastfeeding
C = Cost of treating x

In order to calculate the cost savings using the Disease-based model (B_D), estimates of disease occurrence and estimates of reduction that could be expected from full breastfeeding for 12 weeks were developed based on existing published data. Incidence of cause-specific infant illness is not available, therefore estimates of morbidity were based on published data for under 15-year-olds and 1-4-year-olds and adjusted. This will yield a very low estimate, since disease incidence decreases with age during childhood; therefore a factor of 4 is used as a multiplier to estimate the incidence in infants. Based on the illnesses identified in the introduction and the relative risks gleaned from the same literature, it is estimated that rates of hospitalizations for infectious disease is approximately 167.9 per 10,000; however, the incidence of non-hospitalized infectious disease is easily ten to 15 times as high (estimated factor = 12.5). Infectious disease incidence is cut in half by full breastfeeding. Malignant neoplasia (9.5 per 10,000) is also reduced by at least one sixth and chronic gastrointestinal problems (44.3 per 10,000) are reduced by about 25%. In addition, insulin dependent diabetes among children under 15 years of age (1.5/10,000) is halved by breastfeeding. The average cost of an incidence of infectious disease, including both severe and mild, is $600, while the treatment of the first year of cancer is estimated at $28,500, and the annual excess cost of treating diabetes is approximately $7,500. Therefore, with a conservative assumption that neoplasia demands two years of care, chronic gastrointestinal disease demands 5 years of care, and diabetes would demand 20 years, the Disease-based Model yields a benefit of $4.294 billion.

Disease-based Model Calculation

Benefit (savings) = _ k_x (I_x x R_x x P_x x C_x)

((0.01679 x 4 x 12.5 x 0.5 x 3,800,000 x $600) + 2 (0.00095 x 4 x 12.5 x 0.17 x 3,800,000 x $28,500) + 5(0.00443 x 4 x 12.5 x 0.25 x 3,800,000 x $600)) + 20 (0.00015 x 0.5 x 3,800,000) = $4.294 billion

Infectious disease-only hospitalization model

Using a similar approach and data on hospitalizations for those aged 1–4, there are about 412,000 hospitalizations among 16 million children, or an incidence of 0.025. In this model there is again the assumption that hospitalizations reflect only 1:12.5 episodes of illness and that the rate of illness is three times as high as in infants in this age group. Therefore, with these data, which do not include neoplasia, the Disease-based model for infectious disease hospitalization only yields a benefit of $1.217 billion.

Infectious disease–only hospitalization model calculation

(0.02575 x 3 x 12.5) x 0.5 x 4.2 million x $600 = $1.217 billion

HEALTH EXPENDITURE MODEL

The Health Expenditure Model is based on the amount spent on healthcare among infants (24% of the $50 billion spent on children's healthcare in 1987, or a total, extrapolated from cost projections, of about $24 billion in 1991.)

Benefit (savings) = _ (E x D_X x R_X)

where E = Age-specific expenditure on healthcare

D_X = Percent of costs due to disease x

R_X = Reduction in rate of x associated with breastfeeding

Therefore, the Health Expenditure Model for infectious and neoplastic disease yields a benefit of $3.96 billion

Health Expenditure Model calculations for infectious and neoplastic disease

Benefit (savings) = _ (E x D_X x R_X)

($24 billion x 0.32 x 0.5) + ($24 billion x 0.02 x 0.25) = $3.96 billion

HOUSEHOLD EXPENSE MODEL

Benefit (savings) = P _ (F + S + V - N)

where P = Population at risk of x, or number of live births

F = Cost of formula for three months, at about $170 a month

S = Cost of family planning commodities for three months, at about $33 per month

V = Cost of two visits to healthcare provider, at about $60. each

N = Cost of extra maternal nutritional/caloric intake, at about 50¢ a day

The Household Expense Model includes the costs of formula and family planning, as well as a factor for decreased health expenditures extrapolated from earlier studies35, yielding a benefit of $2.835 billion, or $2.331 if you assume the health system's costs to be covered.

Household Expense Model Calculation

Benefit (savings) = P _ (F + S + V - N)
(4.2 million)($500 + $100 + $120 - $45) = $2.835 billion, or $2.331 if it is assumed that all healthcare costs are covered

COST BENEFIT ANALYSIS MODEL

A Cost Benefit calculation is used to assess savings or losses associated with breastfeeding over the next ten years. Keeping the dollar constant, the model is:

$\_Bi/(1 + r)^i - \_Ci/(1 + r)^i$

where B = Benefits (savings),
r = Rate at which the value of the dollar falls, assuming no inflation
C = Costs

However, since there are no capitol costs in these calculations, with the exception of the very small amount needed for lactation consultant training, we assume the denominators to be equal. Therefore, the equation used is simply _B - _C, or may be presented as a ratio, C/B.

Appendix 2: Breastfeeding Resource List

by Cynthia Good Mojab, M.S.

Each year new research expands our understanding of breastfeeding, human lactation, and the needs of breastfeeding mothers and children in diverse situations around the world. The "Breastfeeding Resource List" reflects this dynamic process, and it will evolve with each edition of *Breastfeeding Annual International*. The best breastfeeding resources are dynamic, too, as they change to incorporate new evidence-based information and practices and to overcome cultural, economic and political barriers to breastfeeding. The quality of the resources included here necessarily varies in reflection of this process.

This list is but a sampling of the many breastfeeding resources available today; more entries will be added in the next edition. It is organized into three major sections: Resources for Lactation and Other Health Professionals, Advocacy and Social Marketing Resources, and Resources for Parents. However, readers may find helpful information in any section of the list. Books, periodicals and other publications, multimedia resources, organizations and Internet-based resources are included. Additional resources can be found by searching the Internet, looking for resource lists on the websites of organizations included in this list, or consulting with a reference librarian at a community or university library. Many larger libraries subscribe to electronic databases (accessible from the Internet or on CD-ROM) that can be searched for full-text articles, article abstracts or bibliographic information on articles related to breastfeeding. Many state, national and international departments and agencies of public health offer breastfeeding resources, as well.

When considering the breastfeeding information and support offered by an organization in a publication, or in another resource, critical thinking is essential. For example:

- What are the goals and potential biases of the organization or author?
- Who funded the work and how might their goals and biases have affected it?
- When, where and how was the work conducted? Might it be out-of-date or applicable in only some situations?
- Is the work or publication peer-reviewed?
- Might any conflicts of interest exist?
- Is the information based on opinion, research, personal experience or clinical experience? What are the limitations of the research? Is the experience limited or broad?
- Does the organization or author (or the sponsor or donor) comply with the WHO/UNICEF International Code of Marketing of Breastmilk Substitutes?

Questions such as these will help the consumer judge the quality of the resources as well as their applicability in any given situation.

RESOURCES FOR LACTATION AND OTHER HEALTH PROFESSIONALS

Books

Breastfeeding: A Guide for the Medical Profession
Ruth Lawrence and Robert Lawrence
Mosby Year Book, 1998
Offers comprehensive information on all aspects of breastfeeding of relevance to the medical profession.

Breastfeeding and Human Lactation
Jan Riordan, Ed.D., R.N., I.B.C.L.C., F.A.A.N., and Kathleen Auerbach, Ph.D., I.B.C.L.C.
Jones and Bartlett Publishers, Inc., 1999
Utilizes a strong clinical focus and includes technical know-how, research and news reports.

Breastfeeding: Biocultural Perspectives
Edited by Patricia Stuart-Macadam, Ph.D., and Katherine Dettwyler, Ph.D.
Aldine de Gruyter, 1995
Illustrates the important and complex roles that biology, culture and evolution play in the human behavior of breastfeeding.

Breastfeeding Management in Australia

Edited by Wendy Brodribb

Nursing Mothers' Association of Australia, 1997

Covers the basics of anatomy and physiology, reviews common breastfeeding problems and offers effective management techniques for the antenatal period and early days of breastfeeding.

Breastfeeding the Newborn: Clinical Strategies for Nurses

Marie Biancuzzo

Mosby, Inc., 1999

Helps healthcare professionals provide proper breastfeeding management in a variety of postpartum situations; includes clinical scenarios, interviewing techniques and illustrations.

Clinical Lactation: A Visual Guide

Kathleen Auerbach, Ph.D., I.B.C.L.C., and Jan Riordan, Ed.D., R.N., I.B.C.L.C., F.A.A.N.

Jones and Bartlett Publishers, Inc., 2000

Contains color photographs documenting normal breasts and nipples, as well as genetic anomalies and trauma due to mechanical damage, allergy and disease.

Counseling the Nursing Mother: A Lactation Consultant's Guide

Judith Lauwers and Debbie Shinskie

Jones and Bartlett Publishers, Inc., 2000

Addresses various topics in the field of lactation consulting, including basic anatomy and physiology, breastfeeding techniques, counseling methods and skills, breastfeeding promotion and the professional role of the lactation consultant.

Current Issues in Clinical Lactation 2000

Edited by Kathleen Auerbach, Ph.D., I.B.C.L.C.

Jones and Bartlett Publishers, Inc., 2000

Highlights clinical reports and case series that illustrate particular clinical lactation problems and how they were resolved; published annually.

Drugs in Pregnancy and Lactation: A Reference Guide to Fetal and Neonatal Risk

Gerald Briggs, Roger Freeman and Sumner Yaffe

Lippincott, Williams and Wilkins, 1998

Reviews the effects of over 800 types of drugs on nursing infants.

Handbook of Milk Composition
Edited by Robert Jensen and Marvin Thompson
Academic Press, Inc., 1995

Contains data summarizing information on human and bovine milk, including sampling, storage and composition.

Medications and Mothers' Milk
Thomas W. Hale, Ph.D.
Pharmasoft Medical Publishing, 2000

Provides annually published information on almost 600 drugs, vaccines, viruses and herbal medications and their use in breastfeeding mothers.

Pocket Guide to Breastfeeding and Human Lactation
Jan Riordan, Ed.D., R.N., I.B.C.L.C., F.A.A.N., and Kathleen Auerbach, Ph.D., I.B.C.L.C.
Jones and Bartlett Publishers, Inc., 2000

Covers many breastfeeding topics and includes explanatory visuals and important references; is the companion to the text *Breastfeeding and Human Lactation*,

The Breastfeeding Answer Book
Nancy Mohrbacher, I.B.C.L.C., and Julie Stock, BA, I.B.C.L.C.
La Leche League International, 1997

Explores a broad spectrum of information and deals with a wide variety of breastfeeding questions encountered by lactation professionals and lay breastfeeding counselors.

The Breastfeeding Atlas
Barbara Wilson-Clay, B.S., I.B.C.L.C., and Kay Hoover, M.Ed., I.B.C.L.C.
LactNews Press, 1999

Offers a complete, collection of color photos and referenced text explaining common and uncommon breastfeeding situations.

Periodicals

Breastfeeding Abstracts
La Leche League International (LLLI)

Includes a feature article, abstracts of recently published professional articles regarding breastfeeding and human lactation, bibliographic information for other articles of interest and announcements regarding educational opportunities with LLLI, such as workshops, seminars and conferences; published quarterly. Subscription information: LLLI, PO Box 4079, Schaumburg, IL 60168-4079 USA. Tel: 847-519-7730, fax: 847-519-0035, LLLI@llli.org (eMail).

Breastfeeding Outlook

Presents evidence-based strategies for clinical practice, current research with analyses of the conduct of the studies and answers to questions submitted by readers; published quarterly. Subscription information: *Breastfeeding Outlook*, WMC Worldwide, PO Box 387, Herndon, VA 20172 USA. Fax: 703-758-0891, newsletter@wmc-worldwide.com (eMail), http://www.breastfeedingoutlook.com (website).

Breastfeeding Review

Nursing Mothers' Association of Australia (NMAA)

Includes peer-reviewed articles on human lactation and the management of breastfeeding, including original research, case studies, scientific findings, social and ethical aspects of breastfeeding, reviews and letters; published in March, July and November. Subscription information: NMAA, PO Box 4000, Glen Iris, Victoria 3146 Australia. Tel: 61-3-9885-0855, fax: 61-3-9885-0866, nursingm@nmaa.asn.au (eMail), http://www.nmaa.asn.au (web site).

Journal of Human Lactation

International Lactation Consultant Association (ILCA)

Publishes peer-reviewed original research, commentaries regarding breastfeeding behavior and human lactation, case reports related to the practicing lactation consultant and other health professionals involved with breastfeeding, as well as discussions of the business aspects of lactation consulting; published quarterly. Subscription information: ILCA, 1500 Sunday Drive, Suite 102, Raleigh, NC 27607. Tel: 919-787-5181, fax: 919-787-4916, ilca@erols.com (eMail), http://www.ilca.org/index.html (web site).

Leaven

La Leche League International (LLLI)

Offers a feature article—of interest to lactation consultants and health professionals working with breastfeeding mothers—detailing up-to-date information on an aspect of breastfeeding, human lactation, or a related topic; published bimonthly for active LLL Leaders. Subscription information: LLLI, 1400 N. Meacham Road, PO Box 4079, Schaumburg, IL 60168-4079 USA. Tel: 847-519-7730, fax: 847-519-0035, LLLI@llli.org (eMail).

Other Publications

Breastfeeding and the Use of Human Milk (RE9729)
American Academy of Pediatrics, December 1997
Pediatrics, Volume 100, Number 6, pp. 1035–1039

Summarizes the AAP's position on breastfeeding, including its benefits to the infant, mother and nation; has principles guiding healthcare providers in the initiation and maintenance of breastfeeding and offers ways in which pediatricians can support, promote and protect breastfeeding in individual practices, hospitals, medical schools, communities and the nation. It can be read on-line at http://www.aap.org/policy/re9729.html (website).

Breastfeeding Patterns in the Developing World
Farzaneh Roudi, Diana Cornelius and Virginia Vitzthum

Population Reference Bureau, 1999

Includes information in a wallchart format on breastfeeding patterns, child survival and reproductive health information for more than 90 developing countries, as well as on the benefits of breastfeeding, the Lactational Amenorrhea Method and breastfeeding and HIV/AIDS. It can be viewed on the MEASURE Communication website (http://www.measurecommunication.org/reports/bfwc99/bfwc99.htm).

Lactation Consultant Series I
La Leche League International, 1987

Consists of individually published units that stress the lactation consultant's unique role in supporting the breastfeeding mother in difficult situations, such as relactation and induced lactation, breastfeeding the baby with Down syndrome and breastfeeding premature babies. Available from: LLLI, PO Box 4079, Schaumburg, IL 60168-4079 USA. Tel: 847-519-7730, fax: 847-519-0035, LLLI@llli.org (eMail), http://www.lalecheleague.org (website).

Lactation Consultant Series II

La Leche League International, 1999–present

More individually published units on the lactation consultant's role in supporting the breastfeeding mother in various circumstances. Topics include the effect of labor epidurals on breastfeeding, teens and breastfeeding, mastitis and nurslings with congenital disorders. Available from: LLLI, PO Box 4079, Schaumburg, IL 60168-4079 USA. Tel: 847-519-7730, fax: 847-519-0035, LLLI@llli.org (eMail), http://www.lalecheleague.org (website).

Multimedia

The Breastfeeding Atlas CD-ROM

Barbara Wilson-Clay, B.S., I.B.C.L.C., and Kay Hoover, M.Ed., I.B.C.L.C. LactNews Press, 2000

Includes all 230 photos from *The Breastfeeding Atlas*, as well as an imaging program that coordinates the photos with the text; images can also be viewed individually, imported into presentation software or loaded into an image editor, and may be used without charge in educational presentations.

Tongue-Tie: Impact on Breastfeeding–Complete Management Including Frenotomy

Evelyn Jain, M.D., C.C.F.P., I.B.C.L.C., 1994

Helps the physician to identify tongue-tie and to perform frenotomy; demonstrates a comprehensive method of assessment of the impact of a lingual frenulum on breastfeeding and a follow-up management plan for the lactation consultant. Available from: Lakeview Breastfeeding Clinic, 6628 Crowchild Trail SW, Calgary, Alberta, T3E 5R8 Canada. Tel: 403-249-0130, fax: 403-249-0156, evelyn.jain@home.com (eMail), http://www.drjain.com (website).

Organizations Working Exclusively in Breastfeeding and Human Lactation

Academy of Breastfeeding Medicine (ABM)

ABM Executive Office

PO Box 81323

San Diego, CA 92138 USA
Tel: 877-836-9947 (toll free) or 619-295-0058
Fax: 619-295-0056,
eMail: ABM@bfmed.org
Website: http://www.bfmed.org

A global organization of physicians dedicated to the support, promotion and protection of breastfeeding and human lactation through physician education, expansion of knowledge, facilitation of optimal practices and information exchange.

Bright Future Lactation Resource Centre
Linda Smith, B.S.E., F.A.C.C.E., I.B.C.L.C.
6540 Cedarview Ct.
Dayton, OH 45459-1214 USA Dayton, OH 45
Tel: 937-438-9458
Fax: 937-438-3229
eMail: lindaj@bflrc.com
Website: http://www.bflrc.com

A distribution center for information, education and services related to breastfeeding and lactation management, including professional consultations, lectures, courses, professional coaching, teaching materials, printed materials, promotional items and networking information.

Center for Breastfeeding Information (CBI)
Carol Huotari, CBI Manager
Department of Education
La Leche League International
1400 N. Meacham Road
PO Box 4079
Schaumburg, IL 60168-4079 USA
Tel: 847-519-7730 (ext. 245)
Fax: 847-519-0035
eMail: cbi@llli.org
Website: http://www.lalecheleague.org/cbi/CBI.html

Maintains a collection of books and over 17,000 full-length professional articles on breastfeeding and human lactation and related topics, including those abstracted in *Breastfeeding Abstracts*. An electronic database of bibliographic information on the articles (categorized by subject, date, author and journal) can be searched for free via LLLI's website. Annual subscriptions or assistance with individual searches are also available for a fee. Staff provides services such as telephone consultations, bibliographic lists, research interpretation and referral to other sources of information.

Human Milk Banking Association of North America (HMBANA), Inc.

Mary Rose Tully, President
Director of Lactation Services
UNC Women's Hospital, CB# 7600
101 Manning Dr.
Chapel Hill, NC 27514 USA
Tel: 919-966-3428
Fax: 919-852-0985
eMail: mtully@unch.unc.edu
Website: http://www.hmbana.org

A nonprofit organization representing all North American human milk banks that collect, pasteurize and distribute donated human milk. It reviews and revises guidelines for donor human milk banking practices, provides a forum for information sharing among experts on human milk and lactation, provides information to the medical community, facilitates communication among member banks, encourages research on human milk and its use and acts as a liaison between member milk banks and government regulatory agencies. The HMBANA publishes *Guidelines for the Establishment and Operation of a Donor Human Milk Bank* and *Recommendations for Storage and Handling of Mother's Own Milk for Her Hospitalized Infant*. Contact information for member banks is listed on the website.

International Board of Lactation Consultant Examiners (IBLCE)

International Office
7309 Arlington Blvd., Suite 300
Falls Church, VA 22042-3215 USA
Telephone: 703-560-7330
Fax: 703-560-7332
eMail: iblce@erols.com
Website: http://www.iblce.org

A nonprofit corporation that develops and administers a voluntary certification program for lactation consultants through annual examinations, offered in several languages, at many sites around the world. A list of all currently certified I.B.C.L.C.s registered in the United States can be accessed on-line (http://www.iblce.org/registr2.html). The IBLCE International Office serves the Western Hemisphere and Israel. Contact information for additional offices is listed below.

Asia, the South Pacific, Southern Africa, Great Britain and Ireland:

IBLCE Regional Office in Australia
PO Box 13
South Hobart, TAS 7004 AUSTRALIA
Tel: 61-3-6223-8445
Fax: 61-3-6223-8665
eMail: office@iblce.edu.au
Website: http://www.iblce.edu.au

Europe, the Middle East and North Africa

IBLCE Regional Office in Austria
Steinfeldgasse 11
A-2511 Pfaffstaetten AUSTRIA
Tel: 43-2252-20-65-95
Fax: 43-2252-20-64-87
eMail: office@iblce-europe.org
Website: http://www.iblce-europe.org

International Lactation Consultant Association (ILCA)
1500 Sunday Drive, Suite 102
Raleigh, NC 27607 USA
Tel: 919-787-5181
Fax: 919-787-4916
eMail: ilca@erols.com
Website: www.ilca.org

Promotes the professional development, recognition and advancement of lactation consultants globally for the benefit of breastfeeding women, infants and children, organizes an international breastfeeding conference and produces position papers, reports, the *Journal of Human Lactation*, the *GLOBE* newsletter and other publications.

International Registry for Lactation Research

Thomas W. Hale, Associate Professor of Pediatrics
Texas Tech University School of Medicine
1400 Wallace
Amarillo, TX 79106 USA
Tel: 806-354-5529
Fax: 806-354-5536
eMail: tom@cortex.ama.ttuhsc.edu
Website: http://neonatal.ttuhsc.edu/lactreg

Provides the scientific community with potential volunteers for studying human lactation under special circumstances, such as certain medical conditions, problems with lactation and the use of specific drugs during breastfeeding. This confidential registry includes women who are currently breastfeeding and/or planning to breastfeed after delivery. Medical conditions and syndromes and medications of interest are listed on the website.

International Society for Research in Human Milk and Lactation (ISRHML)

Frank R. Greer, Secretary Treasurer
Meriter Hospital Perinatal Center
202 S. Park Street
Madison, WI 53715 USA
Tel: 608-262-6561
Fax: 608-267-6377
eMail: frgreer@facstaff.wisc.edu
Website: http://www.isrhml.org

A nonprofit organization promoting excellence in research and the dissemination of research findings in the field of human milk and lactation. It holds an annual international conference and publishes related monographs.

Lactation Associates

254 Conant Road
Weston, MA 02193-1756 USA
Tel: 781-893-3553
Fax: 781-893-8608
eMail: Marshalact@aol.com
Website: http://hometown.aol.com/marshalact/lactationassociates/home.html

Provides breastfeeding education and consultation to healthcare professionals, including publications, speaker services and conferences.

Lactation Education Resources

3621 Lido Place
Fairfax, VA 22031 USA
Tel: 703-691-2069
Fax: 703-691-3983
eMail: LERonline@yahoo.com

Provides lactation management training programs and innovative educational materials, including training for those desiring to become a certified lactation consultant and continuing education for those who are certified.

Lactation Resource Centre (LRC)

Nursing Mothers' Association of Australia
PO Box 4000
Glen Iris VIC 3146 Australia
Tel: 61-3-9885-0855
Fax: 61-3-9885-0866
eMail: lrc@nmaa.asn.au
Website: http://www.nmaa.asn.au

Offers a reference library of over 15,000 articles on breastfeeding, a comprehensive book collection on breastfeeding and related topics, a research database, videos for rent, a staff of specialists in breastfeeding and human lactation and a database of LRC materials that can be searched by keyword (through an annual subscription or on a fee-for-service basis).

La Leche League International (LLLI)

1400 N. Meacham Road
PO Box 4079
Schaumburg, IL 60173 USA
Tel: 800-LALECHE (toll free in the US) or 847-519-7730
Fax: 847-519 0035
eMail: llli@llli.org
Website: www.lalecheleague.org

A nonprofit service organization offering information and support worldwide for mothers who breastfeed their babies. The organization provides educational opportunities for healthcare professionals (including an international conference, physician seminars and workshops for lactation consultants), publishes periodicals (*Leaven, New Beginnings* and *Breastfeeding*

Abstracts), books, articles and pamphlets, administers the Breastfeeding Resource Center program, trains Peer Counselors and Peer Counselor Program Administrators and houses the Center for Breastfeeding Information. Approximately 7,100 volunteer accredited breastfeeding counselors (Leaders) facilitate more than 3,000 monthly mother-to-mother breastfeeding support group meetings around the world. The website can be searched for breastfeeding information and LLL Groups around the world.

Nursing Mothers' Association of Australia (NMAA)
PO Box 4000
Glen Iris VIC 3146 Australia
Tel: 61-3-9885-0855
Fax: 61-3-9885-0866
eMail: nursingm@nmaa.asn.au
Website: http://www.nmaa.asn.au

A nonprofit organization promoting, protecting and supporting breastfeeding through services for breastfeeding women and their partners and for health professionals such as doctors, lactation consultants and midwives. It provides breastfeeding information via its Lactation Resource Centre, 1,370 volunteer breastfeeding counselors and over 400 community-based breastfeeding support groups throughout Australia. The organization conducts an international breastfeeding conference, as well as seminars and courses, and publishes periodicals (*NMAA Newsletter* and *Breastfeeding Review*), books and booklets.

Professional Organizations Supportive of Breastfeeding

American Academy of Family Physicians (AAFP)
11400 Tomahawk Creek Parkway
Leawood, KS 66211-2672 USA
Tel: 913-906-6000
eMail: fp@aafp.org
Web: http://www.aafp.org

The US national association of family doctors working to promote and maintain quality comprehensive healthcare for the public. The site has breastfeeding information and can be searched.

American Academy of Pediatrics (AAP)

141 Northwest Point Boulevard
Elk Grove Village, IL 60007-1098 USA
Tel: 847-434-4000
Fax: 847-434-8000
Website: http://www.aap.org

Prepares its members to effectively advocate and provide care for infants, children, adolescents and young adults. Its position on breastfeeding is stated in the 1997 AAP Policy Statement, *Breastfeeding and the Use of Human Milk* (RE9729) (http://www.aap.org/policy/re9729.html). The site can be searched (http://www.aap.org/search/query.htm).

American College of Nurse-Midwives (ACNM)

818 Connecticut Avenue NW, Suite 900
Washington, DC 20006 USA
Tel: 202-728-9860
Fax: 202-728-9897
eMail: info@acnm.org
Website: http://www.midwife.org

Accredits midwifery education programs, promotes and administers continuing education programs, establishes standards of clinical practice, creates liaisons with governmental agencies and conducts research. Its position on breastfeeding can be read on-line (http://www.midwife.org/prof/breast.htm). The site can be searched (http://www.midwife.org/search).

American College of Obstetricians and Gynecologists (ACOG)

409 12th St., SW
PO Box 96920
Washington, DC 20090-6920 USA
eMail: resources@acog.org
Website: http://www.acog.com

Advocates for quality healthcare for women, promotes patient education and involvement in medical care and strives to increase awareness among its members and the public of changing issues in women's healthcare. Publishes a patient education pamphlet, *Breastfeeding Your Baby*. The site can be searched (http://www.acog.com).

American Society of Preventive Oncology (ASPO)

1300 University Ave., Suite 7-C
Madison, WI 53706 USA
Tel: 608-263-6809
Fax: 608-263-4497
eMail: jabowser@facstaff.wisc.edu
Website: http://www.aspo.org

A multi-disciplinary society advocating cancer prevention and control through the promotion of the exchange and dissemination of information, the identification and stimulation of new research areas and support of the implementation evaluation of national, state and local programs and policies in cancer prevention and control.

Association of Women's Health, Obstetric, and Neonatal Nurses (AWHONN)

2000 L Street NW, Suite 740
Washington, DC 20036 USA
Tel: 800-673-8499 (USA) or 800-245-0231 (Canada)
Fax: 202-728-0575
eMail: chrish@awhonn.org
Website: http://www.awhonn.org

Develops nursing guidelines and position statements on women's health, obstetric and neonatal nursing practice issues and publishes the *Journal of Obstetric, Gynecologic and Neonatal Nursing (JOGNN)*, presenting clinical scholarship and original research critical to nursing practice. Three position statements regarding breastfeeding can be read on-line (http://209.236.2.215/new/positionstatements/positionstatements.html). The site can be searched (http://www.awhonn.org).

International Childbirth Education Association, Inc. (ICEA)

PO Box 20048
Minneapolis, MN 55420 USA
Tel: 952-854-8660
Fax: 952-854-8772
eMail: info@icea.org
Website: http://www.icea.org

A nonprofit professional organization supporting educators and other healthcare providers who believe in freedom of choice based on knowledge of alternatives in family-centered maternity and newborn care. It provides professional certification programs, training and continuing education programs and educational resources.

March of Dimes (MOD) Birth Defects Foundation
1275 Mamaroneck Avenue
White Plains, NY 10605 USA
Tel: 888-663-4637
Website: http://www.modimes.org

A nonprofit organization working to reduce birth defects, infant mortality and low birth weight and to increase the number of women getting prenatal care. Its Resource Center provides information and referral services to the public. Nursing module publications include *Breastfeeding the Healthy Newborn: A Nursing Perspective* and *Breastfeeding the Infant with Special Needs*. The site can be searched.

National Association of WIC Directors (NAWD)
2001 S Street, NW, Suite 580
Washington, DC 20009 USA
Tel: 202-232-5492
Fax: 202-387-5281
eMail: members@wicdirectors.org
Website: http://www.wicdirectors.org

A nonprofit membership organization founded in 1983 to support, inspire and empower the WIC community through creativity, teamwork and leadership. NAWD represents the 87 State, Territorial and Native American WIC directors and 2,000 Local Agencies providing service to nearly 7.2 million at-risk women, infants and children in 10,000 WIC clinics nationwide. The Special Supplemental Nutrition Program for Women, Infants and Children (WIC) is a short-term preventive health program for low-income women, infants and children at nutrition-related health risks. WIC promotes breastfeeding and provides breastfeeding education and support.

National Women's Health Information Center (NWHIC)
Office of Women's Health
Department of Health and Human Services
8550 Arlington Blvd., Suite 300
Fairfax, VA 22031 USA
Tel: 1-800-994-9662

Website: http://www.4woman.gov

Provides a gateway to the vast array of federal and other women's health information resources. Its website offers health-related material developed by the Department of Health and Human Services, other Federal agencies and private sector resources, including the *HHS Blueprint for Action on Breastfeeding*.

INTERNET RESOURCES

Birthworks Primal Health Research Data Bank

Website: http://www.birthworks.org/primalhealth/keywords.html

An on-line database of information related to the correlations between the "primal period" (from conception until the first birthday) and health in later life; includes bibliographic data and abstracts of journal articles related to breastfeeding.

BreastEd Online Lactation Studies

Sandpiper Education Pty. Ltd.
PO Box 2405 Chermside Centre
Queensland 4032 Australia.
Tel: 61-7-3263-8127
Fax: 61-7-3862-8651
eMail: admin@BreastEd.com.au
Website: http://www.breastedonline.com

Offers an extensively peer-reviewed series of online interactive professional education courses in breastfeeding and human lactation for those seeking certification or continuing education. The site also offers articles on contemporary breastfeeding issues.

Brian Palmer, DDS, For Better Health Website

Website: http://www.brianpalmerdds.com

A website with slide presentations, articles, links and a list of videos related to oral development and health, such as the article *The Significance of the Delivery System During Infant Feeding and Nurturing*, unequivocally advocating breastfeeding.

Computerized Breast Measurement (CBM) System

Website: http://biochem.uwa.edu.au/PEH/PEHres.html

A website detailing the development of a system that measures breast volume and aids in the understanding of breast physiology. Research findings and information on the development of the CBM System are presented in *Studies on Human Lactation: The Development of the Computerized Breast Measurement System* by Cox, Owens and Hartmann (a full-text article available on the website).

International Pediatric Chat (IPC)

Julius Edlavitch, M.D.
2711 Ottawa Ave. S.
St. Louis Park, MN 55416 USA
eMail: edlav001@tc.umn.edu
Website: http://www.pedschat.org

A federally qualified nonprofit organization of pediatric professionals from 127 countries who use live Internet typing (chat) and voice chat as a means of communicating with one another. IPC supports the Baby-Friendly Hospital Initiative and does not accept funds from formula companies. Weekly chat topics include general pediatrics and breastfeeding. Current session schedules and session archives are posted on the website (http://www.pedschat.org/introsched.htm).

Jan Riordan's Breastfeeding Website

Website: http://home.kscable.com/jriordan/index.html

Provides information regarding an Internet course on breastfeeding, links with other Web lactation-related sites, new research results and Jan Riordan's books on breastfeeding.

LACTNET

eMail: LACTNET-request@PEACH.EASE.LSOFT.COM (for information)
Website: http://peach.ease.lsoft.com/archives/lactnet.html

A lactation information and discussion net list of over 2600 professionals interested in the field of lactation consulting and breastfeeding. Several years of archived messages can be accessed and searched on-line or with eMail commands. To join LACTNET, follow the instructions on the website or send this message to Listserv@peach.ease.lsoft.com (eMail): SUB LACTNET <your_real_name>

LactNews On Line
eMail: barbara@lactnews.com
Website: http://www.lactnews.com

Provides breastfeeding advocates and lactation experts with information about conferences, educational materials and breastfeeding courses. It supports the WHO Code concerning the ethical marketing of human milk substitutes and does not accept postings from organizations or individuals not in compliance with the Code.

PubMed
Website: http://www4.ncbi.nlm.nih.gov/entrez/journals/loftext_noprov.html

An on-line database of full-text articles from over 1800 journals. For some journals, user registration, a subscription fee or some other type of fee may be required to access the full text of articles.

Ted Greiner's Breastfeeding Website
Website: http://www.welcome.to/breastfeeding

A collection of articles on such issues as the needs of working mothers, sustained breastfeeding, increasing the father's involvement, the threat of HIV transfer through human milk, breastfeeding and maternal health and nutrition, breastfeeding promotion, the meaning of "weaning," and the infant food industry.

Thoughts on Breastfeeding by Katherine Dettwyler
Website: http://www.prairienet.org/laleche/dettwyler.html

Compelling commentaries on complex breastfeeding issues from the perspective of an anthropologist. Topics include culture, thumb sucking, the natural age of weaning, informed consent, infant sleep, nursing past infancy and more. Includes supporting references.

ADVOCACY AND SOCIAL MARKETING RESOURCES

Books

Milk, Money & Madness: The Culture and Politics of Breastfeeding
Naomi Baumslag, M.D., M.P.H., and Dia Michels
Bergin & Garvey, 1995

Offers a provocative review of the history, culture, biology and politics of breastfeeding.

The Nature of Birth and Breastfeeding
Michel Odent
Greenwood Publishing Group, 1992
Challenges Western assumptions on childbirth and breastfeeding.

The Politics of Breastfeeding
Gabrielle Palmer
HarperCollins Publishers, Inc., 1998
A classic book in breastfeeding literature challenging the assumptions of a bottle-feeding culture.

Other Publications

Breaking the Rules, Stretching the Rules 1998: A Worldwide Report on Violations of the WHO/UNICEF International Code of Marketing of Breastmilk Substitutes
IBFAN, 1998
Reports violations of the WHO/UNICEF International Code of Marketing of Breastmilk Substitutes and relevant WHO Resolutions revealed during a 31-country survey conducted between January and September 1997. It can be read in full on the IBFAN website. (http://www.ibfan.org/english/codewatch/btr98/btr98index.html).

HHS Blueprint for Action on Breastfeeding
Department of Health and Human Services, Office on Women's Health, 2000
The first comprehensive national framework to promote breastfeeding and optimal breastfeeding practices; developed by health and scientific experts from 14 federal agencies and 23 healthcare professional organizations, including the American Academy of Pediatrics and the American Academy of Family Physicians. The full text is available on the National Women's Health Center's website (http://www.4woman.gov/breastfeeding/index.htm).

Organizations

Baby Friendly USA (BF-USA)
8 Jan Sebastian Way, Unit #22
Sandwich, MA 02563 USA

Tel: 508-888-8092
Fax: 508-888-8050
eMail: info@babyfriendlyusa.org
Website: www.babyfriendlyusa.org

A nonprofit organization that implements the Baby-Friendly Hospital Initiative (BFHI) in the United States. The BFHI is an international program based on the WHO/UNICEF *Ten Steps to Successful Breastfeeding*. Hospitals and birth centers earn the Baby-Friendly Hospital Award upon successful completion of the program's process for developing the optimal environment for promoting, protecting and supporting breastfeeding.

Baby Milk Action (BMA)
23 St. Andrew's Street
Cambridge, CB2 3AX, UK
Tel: 44-1223-464420
Fax: 44-1223-464417
eMail: info@babymilkaction.org
Website: http://www.babymilkaction.org

A nonprofit organization working to halt the unethical promotion of artificial infant feeding and to protect and promote good infant nutrition. A member of IBFAN, BMA produces briefing papers, the *Update* newsletter and *Tip of the Iceberg* reports on the campaign for the ethical marketing of breast milk substitutes.

Best Start Social Marketing (BSSM)
4809 E. Bush Boulevard, Suite 104
Tampa, FL 33617 USA
Tel: 800-277-4975
Fax: 813-971-2280
eMail: jhl@beststartinc.org

A nonprofit social marketing corporation that publishes and develops training, education, outreach and advertising materials, provides technical assistance for organizations developing or enhancing breastfeeding support programs and offers training in the use of social marketing. The USDA and BSSM have launched a large breastfeeding promotion effort called "Loving Support Makes Breastfeeding Work." This WIC National Breastfeeding Promotion Project is appropriate for all mothers and was initially funded by the U.S. Government. BSSM's Clearinghouse offers low-cost videos, public service announcements, billboard signage, brochures and posters. Its website will be launched by the end of 2001.

Geneva Infant Feeding Association (GIFA)
Box 157
1211 Geneva 19 Switzerland
Tel: 41-22-798-9164
Fax: 41-22-798-4443
eMail: info@gifa.org
Website: http://www.gifa.org

A member of IBFAN producing *Breastfeeding Briefs*, a collection of new research findings on breastfeeding available in English, French, Spanish and Portuguese.

Global Participatory Action Research (GLOPAR)
WABA Secretariat
World Alliance for Breastfeeding Action
PO Box 1200
10850 Penang, Malaysia
Tel: 60-4-6584816
Fax: 60-4-6572655
eMail: secr@waba.po.my
Website: http://www.waba.org.br/glopar.htm

Strives to empower national groups and individuals around the world to protect, promote and support breastfeeding, identify key obstacles to breastfeeding, help policymakers, program planners and NGO target strategies to improve breastfeeding, develop materials that measure implementation of the 1990 Innocenti Declaration and of other international policy guidelines.

Infant Feeding Action Coalition (INFACT) Canada
6 Trinity Square
Toronto, Ontario M5G 1B1 Canada
Tel: 416-595-9819
Fax: 416-591-9355
eMail: info@infactcanada.ca
Website: http://www.infactcanada.ca

INFACT is a non-governmental, nonprofit organization that supports and protects breastfeeding in Canada; it is the North American representative for IBFAN. INFACT produces and distributes educational resources, produces a newsletter, monitors and critiques marketing practices of the infant-feeding industry in accordance with the WHO/UNICEF International Code of Marketing of Breast-Milk Substitutes, seeks to influence government policy to protect breastfeeding, promotes and supports the Nestlé boycott, organizes World Breastfeeding Week across Canada and promotes and supports the Baby-Friendly Hospital Initiative.

International Baby Food Action Network (IBFAN)

Website: http://www.ibfan.org

A coalition of more than 150 public interest groups in over 90 developing and industrialized nations. IBFAN works globally to improve the health and well-being of babies and young children, their mothers and their families through the protection, promotion and support of breastfeeding and optimal infant-feeding practices and the elimination of unethical marketing of infant foods, feeding bottles and teats. Contact information for all Regional Coordinating Offices can be found on the IBFAN website (http://www.ibfan.org). A few Regional Coordinating Offices are listed here:

North America

INFACT Canada

10 Trinity Square
Toronto M5G IBI
Ontario PO Box 781Canada
Tel: 416-595-9819
Fax: 416-591-9355
eMail: infact@ftn.net
Website: http://www.infactcanada.ca

Europe

GIFA

PO Box 157
1211 Geneva 19, Switzerland
Tel: 41-22-798-9164
Fax: 41-22-798-4443
eMail: philipec@iprolink.ch

Asia

IBFAN Penang/ICDC
PO Box 19
10700 Penang, Malaysia
Tel: 604-8905799
Fax: 604-8907291

Africa

IBFAN Africa
Centrepoint
Cnr of Tin and Walker Streets
Mbabane, Swaziland
Tel: 268-404-5006
Fax: 268-404-0546
eMail: ibfanswd@realnet.co.sz

Latin America

IBFAN Latin America
25 Av. 2–70 zona 7
Residencias Altamira
Ciudad de Guatemala, Guatemala C.A. CP 01007
Tel/Fax: 502-474-0188
eMail: Ruth.arango@starnet.net.gt
Website: http://yabiru.fmed.uba.ar/ibfan

LINKAGES
Academy for Educational Development
1825 Connecticut Avenue, NW
Washington, DC 20009 USA
Tel: 202-884-8221
Fax: 202-884-8977
eMail: linkages@aed.org
Website: http://www.linkagesproject.org

A global program funded by United States Agency for International Development (USAID) that provides technical assistance to organizations promoting breastfeeding. It is managed by the Academy for Education

Department, which jointly provides program direction and technical leadership with LINKAGES' partners: La Leche League International, Population Services International and Wellstart International. LINKAGES and partners' tools include: a results-oriented methodology for behavior change, mother-to-mother support groups, advocacy and policy analysis materials, evaluation and monitoring instruments and social marketing strategies. It also engages in applied research to identify effective program strategies. The site can be searched (http://linkagesproject.org/search.html).

MEASURE Communication
Population Reference Bureau
1875 Connecticut Avenue, NW, Suite 520
Washington, DC 20009-5728 USA
Tel: 202-483-1100
Fax: 202-328-3937
eMail: popref@prb.org
Website: http://www.measureprogram.org

Funded in 1997 by the United States Agency for International Development (USAID) and implemented by the Population Reference Bureau. Its five projects are dedicated to providing accurate and timely information on population, health and nutrition in developing countries. The projects offer technical services in data collection, analysis, dissemination and use. The website offers reports (http://www.measurecommunication.org/reports), such as *Breastfeeding Patterns in the Developing World*, a wallchart of data on breastfeeding patterns, child survival and reproductive health in 90 developing countries (http://www.measurecommunication.org/reports/bfwc99/bfwc99.htm).

National Alliance for Breastfeeding Advocacy (NABA)
254 Conant Road
Weston, MA 02493-1756 USA
Tel: 781-893-3553
Fax: 781-893-8608
eMail: Marshalact@aol.com
Website: http://hometown.aol.com/marshalact/Naba/home.html

Dedicated to the promotion, protection and support of breastfeeding in the U.S. This IBFAN group coordinates efforts by organizations, institutions, agencies and individuals toward the development of strategic plans, policies and goals for breastfeeding reform. NABA publishes information on breastfeeding advocacy; some publications are free.

National Healthy Mothers, Healthy Babies Coalition (HMHB)
121 North Washington St.
Suite 300
Alexandria, VA 22314 USA
Tel: 703-836-6110
Fax: 703-836-3470
eMail: info@hmhb.org
Website: http://www.hmhb.org

A coalition of over 80 community and national organizations, federal agencies and medical and business associations engaging in public education to improve prenatal care and promote breastfeeding. The HMHB Breastfeeding Promotion Issue Committee educates child, maternal health and business communities about the many benefits of breastfeeding during the first year of life. The Committee's publications include: *What Gives These Companies a Competitive Edge: Worksite Support for Breastfeeding Employees, Establishing a Lactation Room at the Worksite* and *Working and Breastfeeding: Can You Do It? Yes, You Can!*

Population Services International (PSI)
PSI/Washington
1120 19th Street, NW, Suite 600
Washington, DC 20036 USA
Tel: 202-785-0072
Fax: 202-785-0120
eMail: generalinfo@psiwash.org
Website: http://www.psi.org

A nonprofit social marketing organization, develops programs to encourage healthful behavior and increase the availability of health products and services at prices low-income people can afford. In partnership with LINKAGES, PSI promotes improvement in maternal and child nutrition.

Promotion of Mother's Milk, Inc. (ProMoM)
PO Box 3912
New York, NY 10163 USA
Tel: 1-877-645-7666
Fax: 305-252-0419

eMail: info@promom.org
Website: http://www.promom.org

A nonprofit organization dedicated to increasing public awareness and public acceptance of breastfeeding. Its website includes breastfeeding information, reasons to breastfeed, discussion forums (including advice from professionals), suggestions for activism and an art gallery.

United Nations International Children's Fund (UNICEF)

UNICEF House
3 United Nations Plaza
New York, New York 10017 USA
Tel: 212-326-7000
Fax: 212-887-7465 or 212-887-7454
eMail: netmaster@unicef.org
Website: http://www.unicef.org

An integral part of the United Nations system, UNICEF cooperates with national governments, non-governmental organizations and other United Nations agencies in 161 countries and territories as it advocates for the rights of children. Its activities include making pregnancy and childbirth safe, encouraging the care and stimulation that offer the best possible start in life (e.g., breastfeeding), helping prevent childhood illness and death and combatting discrimination and cooperating with communities to ensure that girls as well as boys attend school. UNICEF provides training, programs and a variety of publications and audio-visual materials (http://www.unicef.org/catalogues). The website can be searched (http://www.unicef.org/search/searcnewx.htm).

Wellstart International

4062 First Avenue
San Diego, CA 92103-2045 USA
Tel: 619-295-5192 (information) or 619-295-5193 (breastfeeding help line)
eMail: info@wellstart.org
Website: http://www.wellstart.org

A nonprofit, private organization that promotes, protects and supports optimal infant and maternal health and nutrition. It is a partner of LINKAGES. Wellstart provides breastfeeding and lactation training and materials in English, French and Spanish for students and healthcare providers. Publications include *Lactation Management Self-Study Modules, Lactation Management Curriculum: A Faculty Guide for Schools of Medicine, Nursing, and Nutrition* (4th ed.), *Community-based Breastfeeding Support Trilogy, Tool Kit for Monitoring and Evaluating Breastfeeding Practices and Programs* and *Investing in the Future: Women, Work and Breastfeeding* (video).

Women's Environmental Network (WEN) Trust

PO Box 30626
London E1 1TZ UK
Tel: 0207-481-9004
Fax: 0207-481-9144
eMail: wenuk@gn.apc.org
Website: http://www.gn.apc.org/wen

A registered charity educating, informing and empowering women who care about the environment. It tackles issues of the greatest concern to women by offering support and guidance on how to take positive, practical action at home and in the community. WEN provides online information on topics such as breastfeeding and the environment, breastfeeding and pollution and the duration of breastfeeding (http://www.breastfeeding.co.uk/wen/wen1.html).

World Alliance for Breastfeeding Action (WABA)

PO Box 1200, 10850
Penang, Malaysia
Tel: 60-4-6584816
Fax: 60-4-6572655
eMail: secr@waba.po.my
Website: http://www.waba.org.br

A worldwide network of organizations and individuals who believe breastfeeding is the right of all children and mothers. Its seeks to protect, promote and support this right through various activities, campaigns and programs, such as World Breastfeeding Week, the Global Participatory Action Research (GLOPAR) Project and the International Labor Organization (ILO) Convention Campaign. WABA acts on the Innocenti Declaration and works in conjunction with UNICEF. Materials are available in various languages on the WABA website (http://www.waba.org.br/otherlanguages.htm).

World Health Organization (WHO)

Headquarters Office in Geneva
Avenue Appia 20
1211 Geneva 27, Switzerland
Telephone: 41-22-791-21-11
Fax: 41-22-791-3111
Telex: 415-416
Telegraph: UNISANTE GENEVA
eMail: info@who.int
Website: http://www.who.int

A specialized agency of the United Nations with 191 member states that promotes technical cooperation for health among nations, carries out programs to control and eradicate disease and strives to improve the quality of human life. WHO's long-standing partnership with UNICEF includes the launch of such initiatives as Baby-Friendly Hospitals to promote breast-feeding. The on-line catalogue includes many publications on maternal and child health, including several on support, promotion and protection of breastfeeding (http://www.who.int/dsa/cat98/mat8.htm). The website can be searched (http://chef.who.int:9654/?WHOhq + WHOhqHTML).

Internet Resources

Breastfeeding Committee for Canada (BCC)

Website: http://www.geocities.com/HotSprings/Falls/1136/contents.html

Provides information regarding the promotion of the Baby-Friendly Hospital Initiative (BFHI) in Canada. The BCC provides consultation and expert assistance to hospitals and maternity facilities as they prepare for BFHI assessment process and is developing a plan for the protection, promotion and support of breastfeeding in community healthcare settings.

National Center for Chronic Disease Prevention and Health Promotion Centers for Disease Control and Prevention

Website: http://www.cdc.gov/breastfeeding/support-home.htm

Includes information on breastfeeding promotion and support within the healthcare system, workplace, family and community. Provides links to other resources.

Breastfeeding Resources Website

Division of Nutrition and Physical Activity, Centers for Disease Control and Prevention

Website: http://www.cdc.gov/breastfeeding

Provides information on programs and services currently promoting and supporting breastfeeding within healthcare, worksites and communities around the nation, state legislation regarding breastfeeding and major policies influencing breastfeeding promotion in the U.S.

National Breastfeeding Media Watch Campaign

Bureau of Nutrition Services

Texas Department of Health

Website: http://www.tdh.state.tx.us/lactate/media.htm

Identifies references to breast and formula feeding in all facets of the media (television, advertising, print, radio and film) and works to bring about more positive references to breastfeeding. The website lists contact information for Media Watch coordinators in many states.

Texas Department of Health Breastfeeding Initiative Homepage

Website: http://www.tdh.texas.gov/lactate/bf1.htm

Provides a wealth of breastfeeding resources and information on various breastfeeding programs, such as the Physician Outreach Project, Texas Ten Step Hospital Program and the Mother Friendly Worksite Program.

US Congresswoman Carolyn Maloney's Website

2430 Rayburn House Office Building

Washington, DC 20515 USA

Tel: 202-225-7944

Fax: 202-225-4709

eMail (for constituents): rep.carolyn.maloney@mail.house.gov

eMail (regarding breastfeeding legislation): INTERN4.NY14@mail.house.gov

Website: www.house.gov/maloney

Congresswoman Maloney has introduced several bills supportive of breastfeeding: The Right to Breastfeed Act (passed in 1999), the Pregnancy Discrimination Act Amendment of 1999 (H.R. 1478) and of 2000 (H.R. 3861), The Breastfeeding Promotion and Employers' Tax Incentive Act of 1999 (H.R. 1163), The Breast Pump Safety Act (H.R. 3372) and the Breastfeeding Promotion Act (H.R. 285). Information about breastfeeding and Maloney's breastfeeding bills are included on her website (http://www.house.gov/maloney/issues/breastfeeding/index.htm). A listing of state legislation related to breastfeeding can also be read on-line (http://www.house.gov/maloney/issues/breastfeeding/stateleg.htm). Her site can be searched.

WHO/UNICEF International Code of Marketing of Breastmilk Substitutes
Website: http://www.ibfan.org/english/resource/who/fullcode.html
Provides the full text of the International Code.

Annual Breastfeeding Advocacy Events

World Breastfeeding Week

World Breastfeeding Week (WBW) is celebrated in over 120 countries, usually during August 1–7. WBW is the main global campaign of the World Alliance for Breastfeeding Action (WABA). The theme for 2001, "Breastfeeding in the Information Age," highlights the importance of transforming and conveying the facts of breastfeeding via all the available forms of communication in our era. For more information, contact: WABA Secretariat, WABA, PO Box 1200, 10850 Penang, Malaysia. Tel: 60-4-6584816, Fax: 60-4-6572655, secr@waba.po.my (eMail), http://www.waba.org.br/wbw97/wbw2001.htm (website).

World Walk for Breastfeeding

La Leche League International's World Walk for Breastfeeding celebrates breastfeeding promotion efforts worldwide, brings public attention to the importance of breastfeeding and serves as a fundraising event for the organization. The Walk is held by La Leche League groups globally from May 15 to September 15, often in conjunction with World Breastfeeding Week, August 1–7. Participation is free and open to the public. For more information, contact: Kim Cavaliero, Public Relations Department, La Leche League International, Inc., 1400 N. Meacham Road, PO Box 4079, Schaumburg, IL 60168-4079 USA. Tel: (847-519-7730), ext. 233, Fax: 847-519-0035, PRDept@llli.org (eMail), http://www.lalecheleague.org/llleaderweb/walk.html (website).

RESOURCES FOR PARENTS

Books

Attachment Parenting: Instinctive Care for Your Baby and Young Child
Katie Allison, Allison Granju and Betsy Kennedy
Pocket Books, 1999
Clarifies the benefits of attachment parenting, answers common questions, addresses the options of working parents and lists additional resources.

Bon Appetit, Baby! The Breastfeeding Kit
Elaine Moran
Treasure Chest Publications, 2000
Provides encouragement, support and information for the first six weeks of a baby's life in a journal format.

Breastfeeding: A Mother's Gift
Pamela Wiggins, I.B.C.L.C.
Lactation Associates Publishing Company, 1996
Offers helpful breastfeeding information and techniques for overcoming common breastfeeding problems.

Breastfeeding and Natural Child Spacing: How Ecological Breastfeeding Spaces Babies
Sheila Kippley
Couple to Couple League, 1999
Provides information on the contraceptive effects of breastfeeding based on scientific research and personal experience, including explanations of the difference between "ecological" and "cultural" breastfeeding.

Breastfeeding I Can Do That: A Do It Yourself Guide
Sue Cox
TasLac, 1997
Addresses the basics of breastfeeding, common myths, unusual breastfeeding situations, working and weaning in an easy-to-read style.

Breastfeeding Pure and Simple
Gwen Gotsch
La Leche League International, 2000
Guides mothers through the early months of the nursing relationship.

Breastfeeding the Adopted Baby
Debra Stewart Peterson
Corona Publishing Company, 1999

Offers step-by-step guidance on inducing lactation in a woman who has not given birth.

How Weaning Happens
Diane Bengson
La Leche League International, 2000

Covers questions about the natural process of weaning in a reassuring manner; includes a diverse collection of personal weaning experiences of breastfeeding mothers.

Mothering Multiples: Breastfeeding and Caring for Twins or More!
Karen Gromada
La Leche League International, 1999

Addresses all aspects of mothering multiple babies, including preparing for a multiple birth, coping with newborns in the NICU, establishing a milk supply and caring for toddler multiples.

Mothering Your Nursing Toddler
Norma Jane Bumgarner
La Leche League International, 2000

Provides critical information and support for mothers who breastfeed their children past infancy.

Nursing Mother, Working Mother: The Essential Guide for Breastfeeding and Staying Close to Your Baby After You Return to Work
Gale Pryor
Harvard Common Press, 1997

Addresses planning for and returning to employment, pumping, storing and transporting milk, alternatives to full-time employment, working from home and staying home full-time.

So That's What They're For! Breastfeeding Basics
Janet Tamaro
Adams Media Corporation, 1998

A humorous but factual guide to breastfeeding addressing universal questions, common myths, nursing in public and employed breastfeeding mothers.

The Breastfeeding Book: Everything You Need to Know About Nursing Your Child from Birth Through Weaning
Martha and William Sears
Little Brown and Co., 2000

Covers the benefits of breastfeeding, basic techniques, breast pumps and other nursing technology, fertility and breastfeeding, toddler nursing, weaning and more.

The Complete Book of Breastfeeding
Marvin Eiger and Sally Wendkos Olds
Workman Publishing Company, 1999

Explains and explores all aspects of breastfeeding, including breastfeeding in the early days and weeks, self care, working and breastfeeding, nursing the premature baby, sexuality and breastfeeding and the concerns of fathers.

The Nursing Mother's Guide to Weaning
Kathleen Huggins and Linda Ziedrich
Harvard Common Press, 1994

Helps mothers avoid premature weaning and create a positive weaning experience for themselves and their children.

The Ultimate Breastfeeding Book of Answers: The Most Comprehensive Problem–Solution Guide to Breastfeeding from the Foremost Expert in North America
Jack Newman, M.D., and Teresa Pitman
Prima Communications, Inc., 2000

Provides new information on why breastfeeding is the healthiest option, how to find local help and how to handle common and unusual breastfeeding situations.

The Womanly Art of Breastfeeding
Revised and edited by Gwen Gotsch and Judy Torgus
La Leche League International, 1997

Offers warm support and up-to-date information for nursing mothers; it is *the* classic book on breastfeeding.

Why Should I Nurse My Baby?

Pamela Wiggins, I.B.C.L.C.

Professional Press, 1998

Provides basic guidance for breastfeeding mothers; used by hospitals and health professionals throughout the world.

Periodicals

Mothering

Peggy O'Mara

Provides inspirational and practical information and support for natural family living through articles on parenting, health, birth, pregnancy, breastfeeding, the experience of childhood and the process of learning; published bimonthly. The current issue of *Mothering* can be read on-line (http://www.mothering.com). Subscription information: *Mothering Magazine*, PO Box 1690, Santa Fe, NM 87504 USA. Tel: 800-984-8116 or 760-796-4859, info@mothering.com (eMail), http://www.mothering.com (website).

New Beginnings

La Leche League International (LLLI)

Inspires breastfeeding mothers around the world through breastfeeding and parenting articles, stories, poems and other information; published bimonthly for LLLI members. Available by subscription and in Spanish (*Nuevo Comienzo*). Articles are indexed in LLLI's on-line database of full-text articles and can be read (organized by issue) on-line (http://www.lalecheleague.org/nb.html. Subscription information: La Leche League International, Inc., 1400 N. Meacham Road, PO Box 4079, Schaumburg, IL 60168-4079 USA. Tel: 847-519-7730, fax: 847-519-0035, LLLI@llli.org (eMail).

The Compleat Mother Magazine

A magazine of pregnancy, childbirth and breastfeeding offering articles and humor promoting natural parenting methods; published quarterly. Subscription information: Greg Cryns, The Compleat Mother Magazine, 5703 Hillcrest, Richmond, IL 60071 USA. Tel: 815-678-7531, greg@rsg.org (eMail), http://www.compleatmother.com (website).

Other Publications

Approaches to Weaning
Nancy Mohrbacher
La Leche League International, 1995
Provides information for breastfeeding mothers trying to decide when and how to wean (pamphlet).

Breastfeeding a Baby with Down Syndrome
La Leche League International, 1997
Offers support and information for the mother breastfeeding a baby with Down syndrome (pamphlet).

Breastfeeding and Sexuality
Esther Schiedel and Marina Chiono
La Leche League International, 2000
Discusses media and cultural images about women's bodies, postpartum body changes, breastfeeding in public, breastfeeding toddlers and sexual relationships (pamphlet).

Common Breastfeeding Myths
Lisa Marasco
La Leche League International, 1998
Tells the well-referenced truth about 24 breastfeeding myths on topics such as the frequency of nursing, infant sleep and nipple confusion (pamphlet).

Nursing a Baby with Cleft Lip or Palate
Nancy Mohrbacher
La Leche League International, 1996
Contains information on the advantages of breastfeeding a baby with a cleft lip or palate, as well as special techniques and advice on breastfeeding after cleft repair surgery (pamphlet).

Sex and the Breastfeeding Woman
Nursing Mothers' Association of Australia, 1997
Offers a frank and informative look at changes in the life and sex life of breastfeeding mothers, including suggestions on coping with this phase of life (booklet).

Organizations

Attachment Parenting International
1508 Clairmont Place
Nashville, TN 37215 USA
Tel/Fax: 615-298-4334
eMail: info@attachmentparenting.org
Web: www.attachmentparenting.org

A nonprofit member organization that networks globally with parents, professionals and organizations, provides assistance in forming attachment parenting support groups and offers educational materials, research information and consultative, referral and speaker services to promote attachment parenting concepts. Information on finding attachment parenting support groups is available on the website.

La Leche League International (LLLI)
1400 N. Meacham Road
PO Box 4079
Schaumburg, IL 60173 USA
Tel: 800-LALECHE (toll free in the US) or 847-519-7730
Fax: 847-519 0035
eMail: llli@llli.org
Website: www.lalecheleague.org

A nonprofit service organization offering information and support worldwide for mothers who breastfeed their babies. The organization provides educational opportunities for healthcare professionals (including an international conference, physician seminars and workshops for lactation consultants); publishes periodicals (*Leaven, New Beginnings* and *Breastfeeding Abstracts*), books, articles and pamphlets; administers the Breastfeeding Resource Center program, trains Peer Counselors and Peer Counselor Program Administrators and houses the Center for Breastfeeding Information. Approximately 7,100 volunteer accredited breastfeeding counselors (Leaders) facilitate more than 3,000 monthly mother-to-mother breastfeeding support group meetings around the world. The website can be searched for breastfeeding information and LLL Groups around the world.

Nursing Mothers' Association of Australia (NMAA)
PO Box 4000
Glen Iris VIC 3146 Australia

Tel: 61-3-9885-0855
Fax: 61-3-9885-0866
eMail: nursingm@nmaa.asn.au
Website: http://www.nmaa.asn.au

A nonprofit organization promoting, protecting and supporting breastfeeding through services for breastfeeding women and their partners and for health professionals such as doctors, lactation consultants and midwives. It provides breastfeeding information via its Lactation Resource Centre, 1370 volunteer breastfeeding counselors and over 400 community-based breastfeeding support groups throughout Australia. The organization conducts an international breastfeeding conference, as well as seminars and courses and publishes periodicals (*NMAA Newsletter and Breastfeeding Review*), books and booklets.

Internet Resources

Adoptive Breastfeeding Resource Website (ABRW)
eMail: naomi@fourfriends.com
Website: http://www.fourfriends.com/abrw

Offers information and support for adoptive mothers interested in breastfeeding. The website includes articles, a message board (with archive), information on support groups, links to other on-line information and recommended reading lists. The website can be searched (http://www.fourfriends.com/abrw/search.htm).

Ammawell
Website: http://msnhomepages.talkcity.com/SupportSt/ammawell

Provides parenting support and information including breastfeeding reading lists, links, advocacy alerts, a breastfeeding art gallery and a list of breastfeeding publications by researcher and author Cynthia Good Mojab, some of which can be read on-line.

Breastfeeding and the Law
Website: http://www.lalecheleague.org/LawMain.html

Essential information on breastfeeding and the law (primarily in the United States), including a link to the article *A Current Summary of Breastfeeding Legislation in the U.S.*

Breastfeeding.com

Website: http://www.breastfeeding.com

Provides a diverse collection of breastfeeding information, including questions and answers, humor, news, breastfeeding advocacy, employment and breastfeeding and message boards and chat rooms. Some of the commercial links from this site violate the WHO/UNICEF Code of Marketing of Breastmilk Substitutes.

Breastfeeding Online

Website: http://www.breastfeedingonline.com

Addresses topics such as the advantages of breastfeeding, breastfeeding and medications, yeast and thrush, advocacy, used breast pumps, eMail lists for mothers and professionals and additional links of interest to breastfeeding mothers.

Breastfeeding Resources

Website: http://www.borstvoeding.com/abon/bf-resources.html

A large collection of links to diverse breastfeeding resources available on the Internet, including sections on frequently asked questions, basic and specific practical breastfeeding information, personal stories, advantages of breastfeeding, activism, information for healthcare providers, information for lactation professionals, attachment parenting resources, breastfeeding and attachment parenting supplies, mailing lists and news groups and organizations.

Empathic Parenting Online Parenting Course

Website: http://parenting.telecampus.com

Offers free guided study on parenting, including sections on birth, breastfeeding, separation, the family bed, baby weaning, the influence of a parent's upbringing on their care of their own children, the development of the brain and the influence of culture.

Jane's Breastfeeding and Childbirth Resources

Website: http://www.breastfeeding.co.uk

Serves as a gateway to pregnancy, childbirth and breastfeeding information, including breastfeeding articles, discussion forums, over 150 links to breastfeeding resources and the Women's Environmental Network Trust's web pages on breastfeeding (http://www.breastfeeding.co.uk/wen/wen1.html).

Lactational Amenorrhea Resources

Website: http://www.nd.edu/~mmeineke/kelly/lam/lam.html

Provides on-line resources for those who are experiencing lactational amenorrhea and/or wish to use lactational amenorrhea to postpone pregnancy. Includes frequently asked questions, eMail lists, publication lists and links.

Lactations: Daily Inspiration for the Nursing Mother

Website: http://www.lactations.com

Offers a diverse collection of thoughts, wisdom and encouragement on the breastfeeding relationship and its benefits, as well as a bulletin board and links.

Lactivist

eMail: lactivist@lactivist.com

Website: http://www.lactivist.com

Provides information on how to breastfeed, offers solutions for breastfeeding problems, discusses contemporary issues in breastfeeding and provides links to breastfeeding resources. It also has a message board and several eMail lists, including one for adoptive breastfeeding mothers.

Online Breastfeeding Help Form

La Leche League International

Website: http://www.lalecheleague.org/helpform.html

Permits breastfeeding mothers to electronically submit a detailed question to an accredited La Leche League Leader who will reply by eMail within a week. Questions may be submitted in English, Spanish, German, Italian or Japanese.

Mothering Your Nursing Toddler

Website: http://www.myntoddler.com

Offers information on Norma Jane Bumgarner's book, as well as a collection of comments and input from readers on various topics related to breastfeeding past infancy.

Parent Soup's La Leche League (LLL) Areas

Website: http://www.parentsoup.com/library/laleche.html

Website: http://www.parentsoup.com/experts/leche.html

Offers information in their library about LLL, as well as breastfeeding information produced by LLL. Parent Soup also hosts a La Leche League question-and-answer area.

Mothering Discussion Boards

eMail: webmaster@mothering.com

Website: http://www.mothering.com

Allows parents to share their experiences in moderated discussions regarding pregnancy, birth, breastfeeding, family living, health and education; hosted by *Mothering* magazine.

Natural Child Project

Website: http://www.naturalchild.org

Offers articles, parenting advice, an attachment parenting family directory, links and reviews of other parenting sites, a children's art gallery and much more.

The Breastfeeding Ring

Website: http://nav.webring.yahoo.com/hub?ring=bfing&list

Provides links to websites related to breastfeeding, as well as natural parenting, pregnancy and birth.

Cynthia Good Mojab, M.S. Clinical Psychology, is a private researcher and author specializing in the areas of psychology, culture and the family. She has authored numerous publications on breastfeeding, works as Research Associate in the Publications Department of a Leche League International and has been a La Leche League Leader since 1998. Her website, Ammawell, provides breastfeeding and parenting information and support.

Appendix 3: A Current Summary of Breastfeeding Legislation in the U.S.

By Elizabeth N. Baldwin, Esq., and Kenneth A. Friedman, Esq.

As of May, 2001

BREASTFEEDING LEGISLATION: IN GENERAL

Breastfeeding legislation has been enacted in over one-half of the United States. Initially, legislation concerned itself with breastfeeding in public issues, clarifying that mothers have a right to breastfeed where they go with their baby. Since then, other issues have arisen, such as exempting breastfeeding mothers from jury duty, or protecting breastfeeding mothers when they return to work. A few states have enacted laws that require courts in family law cases (divorce or separation) to consider breastfeeding in making custody and visitation or parenting time decisions. Two states exempt mothers nursing their children in their cars from the seatbelt laws. Maryland became the first state to provide an exemption from the sales tax laws for breastfeeding accessories, such as pumps, shields, and other items that are used by breastfeeding mothers.

This article discusses the current status of breastfeeding legislation, and how it affects breastfeeding mothers. We look at the importance of breastfeeding, and how it affects each of the areas of the law, as well as how mothers can use this information if they encounter problems. Note that a complete listing of all the states that we know of that have legislation, including the language from their laws, is at the end of this article. For information on enacting breastfeeding legislation, see .

IMPORTANCE OF BREASTFEEDING

Breastfeeding is no longer considered to be a lifestyle choice, but a significant health and medical choice for both the mother and baby. As the American Academy of Pediatrics has stated in its new recommendations issued in December of 1997:

> "Research in the United States, Canada, Europe, and other developed countries, among predominately middle-class populations, provides strong evidence that human milk feeding decreases the incidence

> and/or severity of diarrhea, lower respiratory inflection, otitis media, bacteremia, bacterial meningitis, botulism, urinary tract infection, and necrotizing enterocolitis. There are a number of studies that show a possible protective effect of human milk feeding against sudden death syndrome, insulin-dependent diabetes mellitus, Crohn's disease, ulcerative colitis, lymphoma, allergic diseases, and other chronic digestive diseases. Breastfeeding has also been related to possible enhancement of cognitive development." American Academy of Pediatrics, Work Group on Breastfeeding, "Breastfeeding and the Use of Human Milk", *Pediatrics*, Vol. 100 No. 6, December 1997.

> UNICEF and the World Health Organization recognize the importance of breastfeeding through age two and beyond. The Innocenti Declaration, sponsored by UNICEF and WHO, and adopted by 32 governments worldwide and 10 United Nations agencies, states: "As a global goal for optimal maternal and child health and nutrition, all women should be enabled to practice exclusive breastfeeding and all infants should be fed exclusively on breast milk from birth to four to six months of age. Thereafter, children should continue to breastfeed while receiving appropriate and adequate complementary foods for up to two years of age or beyond." *Innocenti Declaration on the Protection, Promotion and Support of Breastfeeding*, 1990.

UNICEF has taken steps to encourage physicians to promote breastfeeding, as set forth in former Executive Director James P. Grant's "Call to Physicians for Support" in 1994. He points out that although physicians have long known that breastfeeding is best for babies, there is now increasing awareness that breastfeeding plays a far more crucial role in the survival and healthy development of children in both industrialized and developing countries alike, than the medical profession ever before imagined. "Study after study now shows, for example, that babies who are not breastfed have higher rates of death, meningitis, childhood leukemia and other cancers, diabetes, respiratory illnesses, bacterial and viral infections, diarrhoeal diseases, otitis media, allergies, obesity and developmental delays. Women who do not breastfeed demonstrate a higher risk for breast and ovarian cancers." J.Grant, "Call to Physicians for Support", published in the July/August 1994 issue of the *Baby-Friendly Hospital Initiative Newsletter.*

More and more studies document the significant health benefits, including increased IQ, and the longer that women breastfeed, the more benefit to them and their children. For instance, a recent study from China indicates that a woman's risk of both pre and post menopausal breast cancer is reduced by 50% if she breastfeeds her children for at least two years. Many people in our society are finally realizing that there are economic as well as medical benefits if breastfeeding is promoted. Hundreds of millions of dollars could be saved if more women would breastfeed, and the US government did not have to purchase such large amounts of artificial baby milk for WIC participants, as well as absorb the cost of increased medical expenses for both mother and baby. It is for these reasons that laws have been passed that encourage women to breastfeed, as it benefits all of our society.

BREASTFEEDING IN PUBLIC

Mothers have a right to breastfeed where they go with their baby, even if that is out in public. It does not matter whether the mother goes to a public or a private place, or even whether they are in a state with legislation. No one has the right to tell a mother how to feed her baby, especially a way that increases the risk of illness to both mother and baby! Legislation has been enacted in nearly one-half of the states in the U.S. because they want to clarify this right, and in some cases, provide a remedy for mothers told to stop breastfeeding. It is hoped that legislation will help to change society's attitudes that breastfeeding is something indecent and should not be done in public. Underlying this, is the goal to increase the rates and duration of breastfeeding recognizing that this is an important health choice that must be encouraged.

Babies need to be breastfed on demand, and mothers should not feel pressured to use bottles. According to the American Academy of Pediatrics, babies do not need to have bottles or pacifiers, and even if a mother wants to use these, they are contraindicated until breastfeeding is well established. Early introduction of bottles or pacifiers can put the breastfeeding relationship at risk, as the baby can develop nipple or bottle confusion, often resulting in the baby not being able to correctly nurse. If this happens, the baby may wean, or have such serious difficulties that the mother may need to seek professional help. Would we want even one mother or baby to have an increased risk of illness just because someone doesn't want to see it? Also, using bottles takes away from the convenience of breastfeeding, as the breast it is always ready and available, at the perfect temperature, with no preparation needed. No breastfeeding mother should be told that she should have to use bottles, anymore than a bottle feeding mother should be told that she should be breastfeeding. Breastfeeding is an act of nurture, not something to be hidden. Mothers should be allowed to choose for themselves how they want to feed their baby, and our society should not discourage their choice, especially when it is one that benefits all of us.

It is important to remember that women have a right to breastfeed in public whether there is a law or not. The purpose of legislation is NOT to legalize it, but to clarify the fact the fact that women have the right to breastfeed in public, or that it is not a criminal offense, such as indecent exposure. Thus, if you are in a state that does not have legislation, you still have the right to feed your baby where you go. Breastfeeding legislation often exempts breastfeeding from any criminal statutes, such as amending an indecent exposure or nudity law. More progressive legislation creates a new law that sets forth a woman's right to breastfeed. Some of the laws provide mothers with legal recourse if they are told to stop breastfeeding, such as New York, which has the strongest law in the nation, where a right to breastfeed as one of a person's civil rights was created.

Not only have states enacted legislation, but various cities and counties have amended ordinances, or enacted laws that protect breastfeeding. One of the most notable is the City of Philadelphia, which submitted an ordinance in 1996 that not only prohibited discriminating against breastfeeding mothers, but also prohibited segregating breastfeeding mothers. In response to other states considering allowing establishments to tell mothers where they can breastfeed, they enacted this law to make it clear that such acts are segregation. In 1999, a federal law was enacted that ensures a woman's right to breastfeed her child anywhere on federal property that she has a right to be with her child. As the legal system continues to recognize and encourage breastfeeding, a message is sent to the public at large that breastfeeding is an important issue; one that has an impact on our lives and the futures of our children. But society's views and taboos are not easily changed. Legislation that recognizes the importance of breastfeeding is just one step toward helping our society become more supportive of breastfeeding.

Frequently Asked Questions

*** I am in a state with no breastfeeding legislation. Do I have the right to breastfeed in public?**

Answer: Yes. The purpose of legislation is to clarify that it is legal, and to change society's attitudes about breastfeeding. As a general rule of thumb, if you have a right to be somewhere with your baby, and you can feed your baby a bottle, then certainly you have the right to breastfeed.

*** I was asked to stop breastfeeding. What should I do?**

Answer: If you are told to stop breastfeeding, you will have to decide whether you want to try to do something about it at the time, or to leave and take action later. If you decide to try to do something about it at the time, you might ask if you can give your baby a bottle. If you are told that you can, you can gently educate by letting them know that no one has the right to tell you how to feed your baby. If you are in a state that has legislation, let them know that there is a law that protects your right. If the establishment is not willing to bend, consider leaving and educating them later on. It is not worth a scene to try to enforce your right, and the upset that may result is not good for mom or baby!

If you are looking at how to handle it after the fact, look at the best way to educate those involved. If you are in a state with legislation, the first step is to give them information about the laws, as well as about the importance of breastfeeding. If your state does not have any legislation, that does not mean you can't breastfeed! However, as you will not have any legislation to educate them with, consider using other states legislation. In all instances, feel free to use this legislation article (as well as the others written by me), as well as other materials showing what an important health choice this is.

If you think you might want to take legal action against the establishment, we recommend that you consult with an attorney to determine your legal rights. Don't forget to visit the American Academy of Pediatrics' site and print out a copy of their recommendations (Nothing sets forth the importance of breastfeeding better than these recommendations! Feel free to contact your for assistance with this. She can help you look at these issues.

*** My state is considering enacting breastfeeding legislation. Is all breastfeeding legislation good, or are there certain types that should be avoided?**

Answer: Not all breastfeeding legislation is positive. Any legislation that restricts or takes away the right to breastfeed should not be supported, and if it has already been enacted, steps should be taken to amend the statute taking out the restriction. For instance, Georgia and Missouri enacted laws trying to support breastfeeding mothers in public, but put restrictions on it requiring the mother to be discrete. This comes from a misconception that if discretion is not required, that there will be problems with women exposing themselves. Yet, the purpose of legislation is to try to change these outdated views about breastfeeding, and encourage more women to make this healthy choice. Thus, such language has a chilling effect on mothers, and is not encouragement, and would authorize anyone who didn't think it was discreet enough to throw the mother out. This is why many of the states provided that a woman has a right to breastfeed even if there is exposure during or incidental to breastfeeding. Recognizing this, Georgia has submitted a bill that would delete this restrictive language.

If your state is considering legislation, make sure no restrictions are included. Remember that Liz Baldwin will be happy to look at any proposed legislation, and assist in the process.

JURY DUTY

Recognizing how difficult it could be for a breastfeeding mother to be called for jury duty, four states have enacted laws exempting such mothers. If you live in California, Oregon, Iowa and Idaho, look at the language of their laws to see if they might apply to you. If you are in another state, there is still much you can do. Consider looking for other exemptions that could apply to you, such as an exemption for parents at home with a child under a certain age (such as Florida, age six), or a general hardship hardship exemption. Information about the effect on your body if you cannot breastfeed or express milk may help them to understand the situation, such as leaking milk, breast infections and abscesses. This may be more convincing than focusing on how the baby will miss you! Consider getting a letter from your baby's pediatrician setting forth how important it is that you be able to breastfeed and not have long separations from your baby.

EMPLOYMENT SITUATIONS

Mothers who want to continue breastfeeding when they return to work may have a difficult situation on their hands, especially if there is no convenient place to express milk, or if their employer is not supportive of this health choice. As a result, several states have looked at trying to encourage employers to support breastfeeding mothers, and three states mandates that all employers do so.

If you live in Minnesota, Hawaii or Tennessee, look at the language of your law, as employers there are required to accommodate breastfeeding mothers who return to work. Illinois just passed a similar law, but it has not yet been signed by the Governor. When it is, Illinois employees will also be protected. Other states consider it important enough to encourage it through legislation, but do not mandate it. For instance, California enacted a very positive and detailed Assembly Concurrent Resolution that contains important information about the importance of breastfeeding when mothers return to work, as well as encouragement of the public and private sector to support breastfeeding mothers. Georgia provides that employers can accommodate breastfeeding mothers. Texas and Florida set up projects to determine breastfeeding policies for state employees. While these projects have not resulted in laws requiring this for their state employees, it makes a strong statement to the private sector to consider this as a health choice. Texas did set up an incentive program for private employers, in that they can advertise themselves as 'motherfriendly' if they adopt the policies set up by the state. More and more states are looking at the best way to encourage mothers to keep breastfeeding when they return to work, as it benefits not only the individual mother and baby, but the employer as well.

Studies indicate that women who continue to breastfeed once returning to work miss less time from work because of baby-related illnesses, and have shorter absences when they do miss work, compared with women who do not breastfeed. (See "Comparison of Maternal Absenteeism and Infant Illness Rates Among Breastfeeding and Formula-feeding Women in Two Corporations" by Rona Cohen, Marsha B. Mrtek, and Robert G. Mrtek, published in the *American Journal of Health Promotion*, Nov/Dec 1995, Vol. 10, No. 2.) Another study indicates that worksite lactation programs can increase breastfeeding rates among employed women to a level comparable to rates among women not employed outside the home. (See "The Impact of Two Corporate Lactation Programs on the Incidence and Duration of Breast-Feeding by Employed Mothers" by Rona Cohen and Marsha B. Mrtek; *American Journal of Health Promotion*, July/August 1994, Vol. 8 No. 6.).

U.S. Congresswoman Carolyn Maloney (N.Y.) drafted a federal bill, previously entitled "New Mothers' Breastfeeding Promotion and Protection Act". This bill, which supports breastfeeding by new mothers and encourages employers to support workplace lactation programs, has been resubmitted as separate bills to Congress. If passed, these bills would provide a tax credit for employers who set up a lactation location, purchase or rent lactation or lactation related equipment, hire a health professional, or otherwise promote a lactation-friendly environment; would clarify the Pregnancy Discrimination Act to ensure that breastfeeding is protected under civil rights law; would require the FDA to develop minimum quality standards for breast pumps. Note that the section that provided mothers with unpaid break time to breastfeed has not been resubmitted. There was too much controversy about this portion of the bill, and it is feared that this might undermine the other portions that have a better chance of being passed.

If you are having an employment problem, consider trying to educate your employer with how it benefits them as much as you and the baby. Look at the illnesses that breastfeeding reduces the risk of, and see if any of these are in your or the baby's father's family. If so, don't hesitate to emphasize how important it is that you breastfeed. Look at practical solutions that can work. Some mothers may benefit from discussing it ahead of time with their employer, and others may decide it is better to say nothing, and just pump when they return to work. Look at where you could express milk in privacy, as well as how much time to you really need to express. Is it possible to use your regular breaks to pump? If so, your situation may be easier to resolve, as your employer may not have any right to tell you what you do on your breaks! If it is taking you more than 15 minutes to pump, or if you feel the separations to work are affecting your milk supply, get some breastfeeding help. Contact your local La Leche League Leader, or a lactation specialist for help in deciding what pump to use, how to use it, and how to maintain your milk supply.

If it looks as if you might end up fired or needing to sue your employer, consult with an attorney right away to learn what time frames you are working under. There can be strict time limits on the filing of lawsuits, and it is important to know what those time limits are.

In any case, feel proud of yourself, that you want to be the best mommy you can, and also a good employee!

FAMILY LAW

To date, we know of three states that require courts to consider breastfeeding of a baby as a factor in determining custody and visitation decisions, including parenting time, namely Utah, Michigan and Maine. Also note that Utah and many other states or counties have specific guidelines designed for children under the age of five that do not call for overnights until 18 months to two years of age.

Note that generally, courts recognize that breastfeeding is important and best for a child, but that the public policy of many states is to focus on how both parents can be significantly involved with their child's life. Thus, if the courts feel they are forced to pick breastfeeding over the father's bond, they are likely to pick the father's bond. Mothers fare much better when they focus on how their child can continue breastfeeding, and also have a significant relationship with Dad. Although many people may think that breastfeeding is inconsistent with Dad having a bond, this is just not true! There are many ways to fashion parenting time so that both objectives can be met.

Address the concerns that arise, such as how Dad can have a significant bond, and breastfeeding can continue. Present choices that are realistic and practical. Look at how to make visitation work, rather than using it as an excuse to restrict the father's access. Feel free to contact La Leche League International for help (or to contact me directly) to discuss any family law case.

CONCLUSION

Breastfeeding legal problems are often solved by education about the importance of breastfeeding. Legislation is one way of showing how important society now views this health choice. Use this information to help you with any breastfeeding legal problems you might encounter.

SUMMARY OF ENACTED BREASTFEEDING LEGISLATION AS OF SEPTEMBER, 2000

ALABAMA: House Bill # 468, 1993

Alabama has no legislation dealing with the right to breastfeed in public, but does have a WIC statute that mentions breastfeeding Code of Ala. § 2212C1 (1999), TITLE 22.

ALASKA: Senate Bill #297, 1998

Amends Section 01.10.060 of the Alaska Statutes to read "In the laws of the state, `lewd conduct,' `lewd touching,' `immoral conduct,' `indecent conduct,' and similar terms do not include the act of a woman breast-feeding a child in a public or private location where the woman and child are otherwise authorized to be. Nothing in this subsection may be construed to authorize an act that is an offense under AS 11.61.123."

Creates a new law, Section 29.25.080 Breast-feeding. "A municipality may not enact an ordinance that prohibits or restricts a woman breast-feeding a child in a public or private location where the woman and child are otherwise authorized to be. In a municipal ordinance, `lewd conduct,' `lewd touching,' `immoral conduct,' `indecent conduct,' and similar terms do not include the act of a woman breast-feeding a child in a public or private location where the woman and child are otherwise authorized to be. Nothing in this section may be construed to authorize an act that is an offense under a municipal ordinance that establishes an offense with elements substantially equivalent to the elements of an offense under AS 11.61.123. This section is applicable to home rule and general law municipalities."

CALIFORNIA Assembly Bill # 1814, 2000

As existing law provides that an eligible person may be excused from jury service only for undue hardship, this bill requires the Judicial Council to adopt a rule of court to specifically allow the mother of a breastfed child to postpone jury duty for a period of one year providing that all steps should be taken to eliminate the need for the mother to physically appear in court to make this request, and providing that at the end of the one year period jury duty may be further postponed upon written request by the mother of a breastfed child. The bill also adds section 210.5 to the Code of Civil Procedure to require that a standardized jury summons would be required to include a specific reference to the rules for breastfeeding mothers. The use of the standardized jury summons shall be voluntary, unless otherwise prescribed by the rules of court.

CALIFORNIA Assembly Concurrent Resolution #155, 1998

This measure "encourages the State of California and California employers to support and encourage the practice of breastfeeding, by striving to accommodate the needs of employees, and by ensuring that employees are provided with adequate facilities for breastfeeding and expressing milk for their children." It also, asks the Governor to "declare by executive order that all State of California employees be provided with adequate facilities for breastfeeding and expressing milk."

CALIFORNIA Assembly Bill #157, 1997

Adds Section 43.3 to the Civil Code, which states "Notwithstanding any other provision of law, a mother may breastfeed her child in any location, public or private, except the private home or residence of another, where the mother and child are authorized to be present."

CALIFORNIA Assembly Bill # 977, 1995

Adds Article 3.35 (creating Sections 319.50 and 319.55) to Chapter 2 of Part 1 of Division 1 of the Health and Safety Code. Requires the State Department of Health Services to "include in its public service campaign the promotion of mothers breast feeding their infants." Also requires, hospitals to make available a breast feeding consultant, or alternatively, "provide information to the mother on where to receive breast feeding information."

CONNECTICUT: Senate Bill #260, 1997

Section 46a-64 of the general statutes is repealed and the following is substituted in lieu thereof "(a) It shall be a discriminatory practice in violation of this section ... (3) for a place of public accommodation, resort or amusement to restrict or limit the right of a mother to breast-feed her child; ... (c) Any person who violates any provision of this section shall be fined not less than twenty-five nor more than one hundred dollars or imprisoned not more than thirty days or both.

Creates a new law that states no person may restrict or limit the right of a mother to breast-feed her child.

DELAWARE: House Bill #31, 1996

Amends Chapter 3, Title 31 of the Delaware Code relating to infant nutrition by creating a new section, 312, which states that notwithstanding any provision of law to the contrary, a mother shall be entitled to breast-feed her baby in any location of a place of public accommodation, wherein the mother is otherwise permitted. The bill contains various preambles that set forth the importance of breastfeeding.

FLORIDA: House Bill #231, 1993

Creates section 383.015 F.S. which states that the breast feeding of a baby is an important and basic act of nurture which must be encouraged in the interests of maternal and child health and family values. A mother may breast feed her baby in any location, public or private, where the mother is otherwise authorized to be, irrespective of whether or not the nipple of the mother's breast is covered during or incidental to the breast feeding.

Amends sections 800.02 (unnatural and lascivious acts), 800.03 (exposure of sexual organs) and 800.04 (Lewd, lascivious or indecent assault or act upon or in the presence of child) to state that a mother's breast feeding of her baby does not under any circumstances violate these sections.

Amends various definition sections of 847.001 by adding the following:

"(3) Harmful to minors: ...A mother's breast feeding of her baby is not under any circumstances 'harmful to minors',"

"(5) Nudity: ...A mother's breast feeding of her baby does not under any circumstance constitute 'nudity', irrespective of whether or not the nipple is covered during or incidental to feeding."

"(7) Obscene: ... A mother's breast feeding of her baby is not under any circumstances 'obscene'."

"(11) Sexual conduct: ... A mother's breast feeding of her baby does not under any circumstances constitute 'sexual conduct'."

FLORIDA: Senate Bill #1668, 1994

Creates section 383.016 of the Florida Statutes which provides for a breast-feeding encouragement policy for facilities providing maternity services and newborn infant care and authorizing use of "baby-friendly" designation. Amends sections 383.015, 383.011, 383.311, and 363.318 of the Florida Statutes relating to breast feeding, administration of maternal and child health programs, education for birth center clients, and postpartum care for birth center clients, to conform, and authorizing a demonstration project on access to breast feeding for public-sector employees. Requires a final report and recommendations to the Governor and Legislature, and provides an appropriation of funds for the project.

Section 6, which creates the demonstration project, states that the Legislature recognizes a mother's responsibility to her job and to her child when she returns to work and acknowledges that a woman's choice to breastfeed benefits the family, society-at-large, and the employer. It establishes an access to breastfeeding for public sector employees demonstration project, which would be conducted to determine the benefits of, potential barriers to, and potential costs of implementing worksite breast feeding support policies for public-sector employees in the state. Written policies supporting breast-feeding practices for the workplace will be developed, which address issues including work schedule flexibility; scheduling breaks and work patterns to provide time for milk expression; provision of accessible locations allowing privacy; access nearby to a clean, safe water source and sink for washing hands and rinsing out any needed breast pumping equipment; and access to hygienic storage alternatives in the workplace for the mother's breast milk.

GEORGIA Senate Bill #29, 1999

Amends Article 1 of Chapter 1 of Title 31 of the Official Code of Georgia Annotated by adding at the end thereof a new Code Section 3119 to read as follows "3119. The breastfeeding of a baby is an important and basic act of nurture to which every baby has a right and which act must be encouraged in the interests of maternal and child health and family values, and in furtherance of this right, a mother may breastfeed her baby in any location, where the mother is otherwise authorized to be, provided the mother acts in a discreet and modest way." Note that Senate Bill 362, 1999 has been submitted to delete the language requiring the breastfeeding mothers act in a discreet and modest way.

Amends Title 34 of the Official Code of Georgia Annotated by adding at the end thereof a new Code Section 3416 to read as follows "3416. (a) As used in this Code section, the term 'employer' means any person or entity that employs one or more employees and shall include the state and its political subdivisions. (b) An employer may provide reasonable unpaid break time each day to an employee who needs to express breast milk for her infant child. The employer may make reasonable efforts to provide a room or other location (in close proximity to the work area), other than a toilet stall, where the employee can express her milk in privacy. The break time shall, if possible, run concurrently with any break time already provided to the employee. An employer is not required to provide break time under this Code section if to do so would unduly disrupt the operations of the employer."

HAWAII House Bill # 266, 1999

Amends Section 378, Hawaii Revised Statutes, by adding a new section to read as follows " [§ 37810.2]. Breastfeeding No employer shall prohibit an employee from expressing breastmilk during any meal period or other break period required by law to be provided by the employer or required by collective bargaining agreement.

Amends Section 3782, Hawaii Revised Statutes, to read as follows "Section 3782 Discriminatory practices made unlawful; offenses defined. It shall be an unlawful discriminatory practice ... (7) For any employer or labor organization to refuse to hire or employ, or to bar or discharge from employment, or withhold pay, demote, or penalize a lactating employee because an employee breastfeeds or expresses milk at the workplace. For purposes of this paragraph, the term "breastfeeds" means the feeding of a child directly from the breast. " It also requires the Hawaii civil rights commission to accumulate, compile, and publish data concerning incidences of discrimination involving breastfeeding or expressing breastmilk in the workplace. The commission shall submit a report to the legislature on its findings no later than twenty days prior to the convening of the 2000 legislature. Nothing in this Act prohibits employers from establishing internal rules and guidelines for employees who may wish to breastfeed or express breastmilk in the workplace.

The preamble to the bill provides

" SECTION 1. The legislature finds that women with infants and toddlers are the fastest growing segment of today's labor force, with at least fifty per cent of pregnant women who are employed returning to work by the time their children are three months old.

The legislature further finds that the American Academy of Pediatrics recommends that women breastfeed for at least the first twelve months of a child's life and urges that arrangements be made to provide for expressing breastmilk if the mother and child are separated.

The legislature further finds that women who wish to continue breastfeeding after returning to work have relatively few needs, such as the availability of suitable, dependable, and efficient breast pumps; a clean, convenient, safe, private, and comfortable location to express milk at the worksite; the opportunity to pump their breasts frequently enough to maintain their milk supply; and an adequate place to temporarily store their expressed milk.

The purpose of this Act is to promote breastfeeding by

(1) Disallowing an employer to prohibit an employee from expressing breastmilk during any meal period or other break period required by law to be provided by the employer or required by collective bargaining agreement;

(2) Prohibiting discriminatory employment practices against women who breastfeed or express milk at the workplace; and

(3) Requiring the Hawaii civil rights commission to compile and publish information on workplace discrimination against lactating employees.

IDAHO: Senate Bill # 1468, 1996

Amends Section 2-209, Idaho Code, relating to Jury Service, to state that the Court shall provide that a mother nursing her child shall have service postponed until she is no longer nursing the child.

IDAHO: Senate Bill # 1115, 1995

Provides an exception to the seat belt law for children under four when the child is removed from the car safety seat and held by the attendant for the purpose of nursing the child or attending the child's other immediate physiological needs.

ILLINOIS: Senate Bill #404, 1997

Amends the Civil Administrative Code by adding Section 55.84 which authorizes The Department of Public Health to "conduct an information campaign for the general public to promote breast feeding of infants by their mothers. ...The information required under this Section may be distributed to the parents or legal custodians of each newborn upon discharge of the infant from a hospital or other health care facility."

ILLINOIS: Senate Bill #190, 1995

Amends Section 11-9 of Chapter 38 the Criminal Code of 1961 the criminal statutes by stating that breast-feeding of infants is not an act of public indecency.

ILLINOIS: Senate Bill # 542, 2001

(Note that this law has been passed by both houses, but has not yet been signed by the governor. It will not become law until this happens.)

Creates the nursing Mothers in the Workplace Act; requires an employer to provide reasonable break time each day to an employee who needs to express breast milk for her infant child; requires an employer to make reasonable efforts to provide a room or location in close proximity to the work area, other than a toilet stall, where the employee can express her milk in privacy.

IOWA: House File #2350, 1994

Amends section 607A.5 of the Iowa Code relating to Jury Service to state that a person shall be excused from jury duty if the person submits written documentation verifying to the court's satisfaction that the person is a mother of a breastfed child and is responsible for the daily care of the child. However, if the person is regularly employed at a location other than the person's household, the person shall not be excused under this section.

IOWA: Senate File # 2302, 1999

Creates a new law, section 135.30A, entitled "Breastfeeding in Public Places" which provides that notwithstanding any other provision of law to the contrary, a woman may breast-feed the woman's own child in any public place where the woman's presence is otherwise authorized.

MAINE: Senate Bill # 888, 1999

An Act to Protect the Health and Wellbeing of a Nursing Infant of Separated or Divorcing Parents. Adds whether the mother is breast-feeding an infant under 1 year of age to the list of factors a judge must consider in deciding parental rights and responsibilities.

MAINE: House Bill # 1039, 2001

Amends the Maine Human Rights Act to declare that a mother has the right to breast feed her baby in any location, whether public or private, as long as she is otherwise authorized to be in that location.

MARYLAND: Senate Bill # 252, 2001

Exempts from the sales and use tax tangible personal property manufactured for the purpose of initiating, supporting or sustaining breast-feeding, including breast pumps, breast pump kits, nipple enhances, breast shields, breast shells, supplemental nursing systems, softcup feeders, feeding tubes, breast milk storage bags, periodontal syringes, finger feeders, haberman feeders, and purified lanolin.

MICHIGAN: Senate Bill # 107-9, 1994

Amends sections 4i and 5h of Act No. 279 of the Public Acts of 1909 to expressly state that public nudity does not include a woman's breastfeeding of a baby whether or not the nipple or areola is exposed during or incidental to the feeding.

MICHIGAN: House Bill # 4064, 1993

Provides in section (6) of § 25.312(7a) of the Michigan statutes that the court may consider whether the child is a nursing child less than 6 months of age, or less than 1 year of age if the child receives substantial nutrition through nursing, as a factor when determining the frequency, duration, and type of parenting time to be granted in family law cases.

MINNESOTA: Senate File # 2751, 1997; 1998 Minnesota Chapter Law 369

Creates a new law under Chapter 181, section 181.939 (entitled "Nursing Mother"), that requires employers to provide reasonable unpaid break time each day to an employee who needs to express breast milk for her infant child. The break time must, if possible, run concurrently with any break time already provided to the employee. An employer is not required to provide break time under this section if to do so would unduly disrupt the operations of the employer.

The employer must make reasonable efforts to provide a room or other location, in close proximity to the work area, other than a toilet stall, where the employee can express her milk in privacy. The employer would be held harmless if reasonable effort has been made.

Amends section 617.23 of the Minnesota statutes to state that it is not a violation of the indecent exposure statute for a woman to breast feed.

MINNESOTA: Senate File # 3346, 1997

Creates a new law, section 145.905 of the Minnesota Statutes, entitled "Location for Breast-Feeding" that provides a mother may breast-feed in any location, public or private, where the mother and child are otherwise authorized to be, irrespective of whether the nipple of the mother's breast is uncovered during or incidental to the breast-feeding.

MISSOURI: Senate Bill # 8, 1999

Creates § 191.915, entitled "Breastfeeding information provided, when, by whom", which requires that hospitals and physicians that provide obstetrical care or gynecological consultation shall provide new mothers and pregnant with information on breastfeeding and the benefits to the child; and with information on local breastfeeding support groups; or offer breastfeeding consultations to new mothers, where appropriate as determined by the attending physician. It also requires the department of health to produce written information on breastfeeding and the health benefits to the child, and to distribute such information to physicians described in subsection 2 of this section and to hospitals and ambulatory surgical centers described in subsection 1 of this section upon request.

Creates section 191.918 of the Missouri Statutes, entitled "Breastfeeding in public permitted" that states notwithstanding any other provision of law to the contrary, a mother may, with as much discretion as possible, breastfeed her child in any public or private location where the mother is otherwise authorized to be. Note that this restrictive language requiring discretion does not promote breastfeeding, and should not be copied by other states.

MONTANA Senate Bill # 398, 1999

Creates a new law under Montana Code Annotated section 50-19-501 which states

"Section 1. Nursing mother and infant protection.

(1) The Montana legislature finds that breastfeeding a baby is an important and basic act of nurturing that must be protected in the interests of maternal and child health and family values. A mother has a right to breastfeed the mother's child in any location, public or private, where the mother and child are otherwise authorized to be present, irrespective of whether or not the mother's breast is covered during or incidental to the breastfeeding.

(2) A unit of local government may not prohibit breastfeeding in public by local ordinance.

(3) The act of breastfeeding may not be considered
(a) a nuisance as provided in Title 27, chapter 30;
(b) indecent exposure as provided for in 455504;
(c) sexual conduct as defined in 455620(1)(f); or
(d) obscenity as provided for in 458201.

The preamble to the bill states

WHEREAS, there are benefits to the child, the mother, and society by encouraging and enabling mothers to breastfeed their children; and
WHEREAS, an infant who is breastfed receives protection against infection, illness, and allergies and longterm positive effects on the development, intelligence, and health of breastfed children have been found; and
WHEREAS, a protective effect against various types of cancer and greater emotional and physical health are found for mothers who breastfeed; and
WHEREAS, breastfeeding promotes sufficient birth spacing, improved vaccine effectiveness, and decreased food and medical expenses, which all have positive societal effects; WHEREAS, the Montana Supplemental Nutrition Program for Women, Infants, and Children (WIC) promotes breastfeeding education and support; and
WHEREAS, legislation to clarify the right to breastfeed is necessary to promote breastfeeding by mothers and remove any stumbling block from influencing a mother's decision to breastfeed or continue breastfeeding out of fear of reprisal.

MONTANA House Joint Resolution # 3, 1991

A joint resolution of the Senate and the House of Representatives of the State of Montana supporting the supplemental food program for women, infants, and children (WIC) to promote breastfeeding in Montana. It provides

"WHEREAS, lactation is an ancient physiological function but has declined in prevalence in recent years; and
WHEREAS, breastfeeding is economical, both medically and fiscally; and
WHEREAS, breastfeeding is convenient and promotes maternal and infant health and the dental health of infants; and
WHEREAS, breast milk provides the best nutrition for human babies; and
WHEREAS, breast milk is unique in providing resistance to disease and protection against allergies; and
WHEREAS, breastfeeding is a high priority health objective for the nation for the year 2000; and
WHEREAS, breastfeeding is acknowledged as giving a baby the best start in life by the American Academy of Pediatrics, the American College of Obstetrics and Gynecology, the American Public Health Association, the National Healthy Mothers/Healthy Babies Coalition, the U.S. Department of Health and Human Services, the Montana Department of Health and Environmental Sciences, and the Montana Public Health Association.

Now, therefore, be it resolved by the Senate and the House of Representatives of the State of Montana

That the 52nd Legislature fully support the stated goal of the Montana Supplemental Food Program for Women, Infants, and Children (WIC) to promote breastfeeding in Montana and to provide consistent and valid education and support so that a woman who chooses to breastfeed her infant is supported in that decision as long as she and the baby desire."

NEVADA: Senate Bill # 317, 1995

Creates a new law (under Ch. 201 of NRS) that states notwithstanding any other provision of law, a mother may breast feed her child in any public or private location where the mother is otherwise authorized to be, irrespective of whether the nipple of the mother's breast is uncovered during or incidental to the breast feeding. This new law also lays out the health benefits to mother and baby, recommendations of AAP, UNICEF and WHO. Also amends criminal statutes (NRS 201.210, 201.220) stating that breast feeding of a child by the child's mother does not constitute an act of open or gross lewdness, or an act of open and indecent or obscene exposure of her body.

NEW HAMPSHIRE House Bill # 441, 1999

Amends RSA 132 by inserting after section 10c the following new section

"13210d Breastfeeding. Breastfeeding a child does not constitute an act of indecent exposure and to restrict or limit the right of a mother to breastfeed her child is discriminatory.

The preamble to the bill provides

I. The general court finds that breastfeeding is the best method of infant nutrition. The American Academy of Pediatrics recommends that children from birth to age one should be breastfed, unless under particular circumstance as is medically inadvisable. WHO and UNICEF have established as one of their goals for the decade the encouragement of breastfeeding.

II The general court finds that medical research shows that human milk and breastfeeding of infants provide many health benefits for a child such as lower rates of death including sudden infant death (SIDS) and decreased incidence and/or severity of diarrhea, respiratory illness, bacterial and viral infections including meningitis, ear infections, urinary tract infections, gastrointestinal infections and chronic digestive diseases, childhood leukemia and other cancers, diabetes, allergies, obesity, and developmental delays. Breastfeeding also provides significant benefits to the health of the mother, including a reduced risk of breast and ovarian cancers, postpartum bleeding, osteoporosis and hip fractures in the postmenopausal period, an earlier return to prepregnant weight, delayed resumption of ovulation with increased child spacing, and the psychological benefit of an enhanced emotional relationship or bonding between mother and child.

III The general court further finds that in addition to the health benefits for mother and child, breastfeeding provides significant social and economic benefits to the state, including reduced health care costs and reduced absenteeism for care attributable to child illness.

IV Therefore, the general court finds that breastfeeding a baby is an important and basic act of nurture that must be encouraged in the interests of maternal and child health and family values.

NEW JERSEY: Senate Bill # 1212, 1997

Creates a new law that provides notwithstanding any provision of law to the contrary, a mother shall be entitled to breast feed her baby in any location of a place of public accommodation, resort or amusement wherein the mother is otherwise permitted. Also provides that the local Board of Health, upon written complaint and having reason to suspect a violation of this act has occurred shall, by written notification, advise the owner, manager or other person having control of the public accommodation, resort or amusement of the initial complaint and of the penalties for any subsequent complaints. Thereupon, any owner, manager or other person having control of the public accommodation, resort or amusement receiving such notice who knowingly fails or refuses to comply with the provisions of this act is subject to a fine not to exceed $25.00 for the first offense following initial notification and not to exceed $100.00 for the second offense and not to exceed $200.00 for each offense thereafter. When there exists no local Board of Health or such board, body or officers having the authority to exercise the functions of the local Board of Health according to law in the municipality in which a violation of this act has allegedly occurred, the state department of health and senior services shall exercise the functions of the local boards of health for purposes of this act.

NEW MEXICO Senate Bill # 545, 1999

Creates a new law, § 28201. [Right to breastfeed.] A mother may breastfeed her child in any location, public or private, where the mother is otherwise authorized to be present.

NEW YORK: Senate Bill # 3999-A, 1994

Creates a new law under the civil rights act (section 79-e) that states notwithstanding any other provision of law, a mother may breast feed her baby in any location, public or private, where the mother is otherwise authorized to be, irrespective of whether or not the nipple of the mother's breast is covered during or incidental to the breast feeding.

NORTH CAROLINA: Gen. Stat. sec. 14-190.9, 1993

In the indecent exposure statutes, it states that notwithstanding any other provision of law, a woman may breast feed in any public or private location where she is otherwise authorized to be, irrespective of whether the nipple of the mother's breast is uncovered during or incidental to the breast feeding.

OREGON Senate Bill # 744, 1999

Creates a new law (Or Rev Stat. 109.001) that provides "A woman may breastfeed her child in a public place."

OREGON Senate Bill # 1304, 1999

Ors 10.050 is amended to read "... (4) a Judge of the Court or Clerk of Court shall excuse a woman from acting as a juror upon the request of the woman if the woman is breastfeeding a child. A request for excuse from jury service under this subsection must be made in writing... (5) Unless the public need for juries in the court outweighs the individual circumstances of the person summoned, a Judge of the Court or Clerk of Court shall excuse a person from acting as a juror upon the request of that person if the person is the sole caregiver for a child or other dependent during the Court's normal hours of operation, the person is unable to afford day care or make other arrangements for the care of the dependent, and the person personally attends to the dependent during the Court's normal hours of operation.

PENNSYLVANIA: PHILADELPHIA

City Ordinance 1996 Amends Section 9-1105 of the Fair Practices Code entitled "Unlawful Public Accommodations Practice" to prohibit a breastfeeding mother from or segregate a breastfeeding mother within any public accommodation where she would otherwise be authorized to be irrespective of whether or not the nipple of the mother's breast is covered during or incidental to breastfeeding.

RHODE ISLAND: Senate Bill # 2319, 1998

Amends Section 11-45-1 of the General Laws in Chapter 11-45 entitled "Disorderly Conduct" to read "In no event shall the provisions of this section be construed to apply to breastfeeding in public."

TENNESSEE Senate Bill # 1856, 1999

Amends Tennessee Code Annotated, Title 50, Chapter 1, Part 3, by adding the following as a new, appropriately designated section Section 5013 (a) An employer shall provide reasonable unpaid break time each day to an employee who needs to express breast milk for her infant child. The break time shall, if possible, run concurrently with any break time already provided to the employee. An employer shall not be required to provide break time under this section if to do so would unduly disrupt the operations of the employer. (b) The employer shall make reasonable efforts to provide a room or other location in close proximity to the work area, other than a toilet stall, where the employee can express her breast milk in privacy. The employer shall be held harmless if reasonable effort has been made to comply with this subsection. (c) For the purposes of this section, "employer" means a person or entity that employs one (1) or more employees and includes the state and its political subdivisions.

TENNESSEE: Tenn. Code Ann. § 559602 (1999)

Provides an exception to the law requiring that all under four (4) years of age in a motor vehicle be properly restrained for a mother from removing the child from the restraint system and holding the child when the mother is nursing the child, or attending to its other physiological needs.

TEXAS: House Bill # 359, 1995

Creates new laws (Subtitle H, Title 2, Health and Safety Code, Chapter 165).

Section 165.001 states that the legislature finds that breast-feeding a baby is an important and basic act of nurture that must be encouraged in the interests of maternal and child health and family values. In compliance with the breast-feeding promotion program established under the federal child nutrition act of 1966 (42 u.s.c. section 1771 et seq.), the legislature recognizes breast-feeding as the best method of infant nutrition.

Section 165.002 states that a mother is entitled to breast-feed her baby in any location in which the mother is authorized to be.

Section 165.003 provides that a business may use the designation "mother-friendly" in its promotional materials if the business develops a policy supporting the practice of worksite breast-feeding that addresses the following: (1) work schedule flexibility, including scheduling breaks and work patterns to provide time for expression of milk; (2) the provision of accessible locations allowing privacy; (3) access nearby to a clean, safe water source and a sink for washing hands and rinsing out any needed breast-pumping equipment; and (4) access to hygienic storage alternatives in the workplace for the mother's breast milk. The business shall submit its breast-feeding policy to the department. The department shall maintain a list of "mother-friendly" businesses covered under this section and shall make the list available for public inspection.

Section 165.004 states that any state agency that administers a program providing maternal or child health services shall provide information that encourages breast-feeding to program participants who are pregnant women or mothers with infants.

Section 165.031 states that the legislature recognizes a mother's responsibility to both her job and her child when she returns to work and acknowledges that a woman's choice to breast-feed benefits the family, the employer, and society.

Section 165.032 sets up a demonstration project to provide access to worksite breast-feeding for department employees who are mothers with infants. The department shall administer the demonstration project and shall determine the benefits of, potential barriers to, and potential costs of implementing worksite breast-feeding support policies for state employees.

Section 165.033 states that the department shall develop recommendations supporting the practice of worksite breast-feeding that address the following: (1) work schedule flexibility, including scheduling breaks and work patterns to provide time for expression of milk; (2) the provision of accessible locations allowing privacy; (3) access nearby to a clean, safe water source and a sink for washing hands and rinsing out any needed breast-pumping equipment; and (4) access to hygienic storage alternatives in the workplace for the mother's breast milk.

Section 165.034 states that the department, if requested by the governor or any member of the legislature, shall submit a report on the demonstration project to the governor or that member of the legislature not later than February 1, 1997. The report must include: (1) a description of the policies developed; (2) a description of the implementation of the policies in Travis County and any problems encountered; (3) the extent of use of any breast-feeding or breast-pumping facilities by department employees; (4) a survey to assess the level of satisfaction with the breast-feeding or breast-pumping facilities and the policies by users and their supervisors; (5) the costs and benefits associated with the demonstration project; (6) a summary of issues raised by employees; and (7) a recommendation of any changes necessary for statewide implementation and strategies for implementing the policies in other state agencies.

UTAH: Senate Bill # 33, 1997

Provides in section 30-4-34 (n) of the statutes for a rebuttable presumption that the visitation guidelines set forth in Section 30333, 30335 and 30335.5 shall be presumed to be in the best interests of the child. It further states that this visitation schedule shall be considered the minimum visitation to which the noncustodial parent and the child shall be entitled unless a parent can establish otherwise by a preponderance of the evidence that more or less visitation should be awarded based upon any of the following criteria, and it specifically lists as a factor the lack of reasonable alternatives to the needs of a nursing child.

Note that Section 30-3-35.5 sets forth a minimum schedule for visitation for children under five years of age. For children under five months of age, it provides for six hours of visitation per week to be divided into three visitation periods in the custodial home, established child care setting, or other environment familiar to the child, and for two hours on holidays. For children 5 - 10 months of age, nine hours of visitation per week divided into three visitation periods in the custodial home, established child care setting, or other environment familiar to the child, and two hours on the holidays. For children from 10-18 months of age, one eight hour visit per week, and one three hour visit per week to be specified by the noncustodial parent or court, and eight hours on the holidays. Phone contact with the noncustodial parent begins at this age at least two times per week. From 18 months until 5 years of age, one weekday evening, and every other weekend from 6:00 p.m. on Friday until 7:00 p.m. on Sunday. From 18 months until 3 years of age, summer visitation shall consist of two one-week periods, separated by at least four weeks, with one week being uninterrupted time for the noncustodial parent, and the remaining week subject to visitation for the custodial parent consistent with the guidelines. The custodial parent shall have an identical one-week period of uninterrupted time for vacation; and brief phone contact with the noncustodial parent at least two times per week. For children three years of age or older, but younger than five years of age, summer visitation is expanded to two two-week periods, separated by at least four weeks, with one two-week period being uninterrupted time for the noncustodial parent, and the remaining two-week period subject to visitation for the custodial parent consistent with these guidelines; and the custodial parent shall have an identical two-week period of uninterrupted time for vacation; and brief phone contact with the noncustodial parent at least two times per week.

UTAH: House Bill # 262, 1995

Amends or creates Sections 10-8-41, 10-8-50, 17-15-25, 76-9-702 and 76-10-1229.5 of the Utah Code to state that a woman's breast feeding, including breast feeding in any place where the woman otherwise may rightfully be, does not under any circumstance constitute a violation, or an obscene, lewd, grossly lewd or indecent act, irrespective of whether or not the breast is covered during or incidental to feeding. Also states that Boards of Commissioners, City Councils of Cities, or County Legislative Bodies may not prohibit a woman's breast feeding in any location where she otherwise may rightfully be, irrespective of whether the breast is uncovered during or incidental to the breastfeeding.

VIRGINIA: Code sec. 18.2-387, 1994

Amends Title 18.2, Chapter 8, Article 5, section 18.2-387 (indecent exposure) of the Va. Code to state that no person shall be deemed to be in violation of this section for breastfeeding a child in any public place or any place where others are present

VIRGINIA: House Joint Resolution #248, 1994

Requests the Dept. of Medical Assistance Services to look at including lactation education and supplies for Medicaid recipients. Sets forth benefits of breastfeeding.

WASHINGTON: House Bill # 1590, 2001

A new section is added to chapter 43.70 RCW to read as follows:

(1) The legislature acknowledges the surgeon general's summons to all sectors of society and government to help redress the low breastfeeding rates and duration in the United States, including the social and workplace factors that can make it difficult for women to breastfeed. The legislature also acknowledges the surgeon general's report on the health and economic importance of breastfeeding which concludes that: (a) Breastfeeding is one of the most important contributors to infant health; (b) Breastfeeding provides a range of benefits for the infant's growth, immunity, and development; and (c) Breastfeeding improves maternal health and contributes economic benefits to the family, health care system, and workplace.

(2) The legislature declares that the achievement of optimal infant and child health, growth, and development requires protection and support for the practice of breastfeeding. The legislature finds that: (a) The American academy of pediatrics recommends exclusive breastfeeding for the first six months of a child's life and breastfeeding with the addition of solid foods to continue for at least twelve months, and that arrangements be made to provide expressed breast milk if the mother and child must separate during the first year. Children should be breastfed or fed expressed breast milk when they show signs of need, rather than according to a set schedule or the location; (b) Breast milk contains all the nutrients a child needs for optimal health, growth, and development, many of which can only be found in breast milk; (c) Research in developed countries provides strong evidence that breastfeeding decreases the incidence and/or severity of diarrhea, lower respiratory tract infection, otitis media, bacteremia, bacterial meningitis, urinary tract infection, and necrotizing enterocolitis. In addition, a number of studies show a possible protective effect of breastfeeding against SIDS, Type I diabetes mellitus, Crohn's disease, lymphoma,ulcerative colitis, and allergic diseases; (d) Studies also indicate health benefits in mothers who breastfeed. Breastfeeding is one of the few ways that mothers may be able to lower their risk of developing breast and ovarian cancer, with benefits proportional to the duration that they are able to breastfeed. In addition, the maternal hormonal changes stimulated by breastfeeding also help the uterus recover faster and minimize the amount of blood mothers lose after birth. Breastfeeding inhibits ovulation and menstrual bleeding, thereby decreasing the risk of anemia and a precipitous subsequent pregnancy. Breastfeeding women also have an earlier return to prepregnancy weight; (e) Approximately two-thirds of women who are employed when they become pregnant return to the work force by the time their children are six months old; (f) Employers benefit when their employees breastfeed. Breastfed infants are sick less often; therefore, maternal absenteeism from work is lower in companies with established lactation programs. In addition, employee medical costs are lower and employee productivity is higher; (g) According to a survey of mothers in Washington, most want to breastfeed but discontinue sooner than they hope, citing lack of societal and workplace support as key factors limiting their ability to breastfeed; (h) Many mothers fear that they are not making enough breastmilk and therefore decrease or discontinue breastfeeding. Frequency of breastfeeding or expressing breast milk is the main regulator of milk supply, such that forcing mothers to go prolonged periods without breastfeeding or expressing breast milk can undermine their ability to maintain breastfeeding; and (i) Maternal stress can physiologically inhibit a mother's ability to produce and let down milk. Mothers report modifiable sources of stress related to breastfeeding,

including lack of protection from harassment and difficulty finding time and an appropriate location to express milk while away from their babies.

(3) The legislature encourages state and local governmental agencies, and private and public sector businesses to consider the benefits of providing convenient, sanitary, safe, and private rooms for mothers to express breast milk.

Amends RCA.88.010 and 1990 c 3 s 904 to exempt the act of breastfeeding or expressing breast milk from the indecent exposure laws.

Creates a new section added to chapter 43.70 RCW to read as follows:

(1) An employer may use the designation "infant-friendly" on its promotional materials if the employer has an approved workplace breastfeeding policy addressing at least the following: (a) Flexible work scheduling, including scheduling breaks and permitting work patterns that provide time for expression of breast milk; (b) A convenient, sanitary, safe, and private location, other than a restroom, allowing privacy for breastfeeding or expressing breast milk; (c) A convenient clean and safe water source with facilities for washing hands and rinsing breast-pumping equipment located in the private location specified in (b) of this subsection; and d) A convenient hygienic refrigerator in the workplace for the mother's breast milk.

(2) Employers seeking approval of a workplace breastfeeding policy must submit the policy to the department of health. The department of health shall review and approve those policies that meet the requirements of this section. The department may directly develop and implement the criteria for "infant-friendly" employers, or contract with a vendor for this purpose.

WISCONSIN: Assembly Bill 154, 1995

Amends and creates sections 948.10, 944.17 (3), 944.20 (2) and 948.10 (2) of the statutes state that the criminal statutes doe not apply to a mother's breast-feeding of her child.

Elizabeth N. Baldwin, and **Kenneth A. Friedman**, are partners in law and in marriage. They are practicing law in Miami, Florida, and consult with parents regarding custody and visitation issues, and conduct family mediation nationwide, including phone mediation. Elizabeth is considered to be the nation's leading expert on breastfeeding and the law, has appeared on numerous television shows, authored many articles with Kenneth, and speaks regularly at conferences and continuing education seminars. Elizabeth is also a La Leche League Leader, and a legal advisor to LLLI. They can be reached at 2020 N.E. 163rd Street, Suite 300, North Miami Beach, FL 33162, 305-944-9100 (Fax 305-949-9029). Ms Baldwin prefers to be contacted by phone or fax.

Index

A Word About Platypus Media from Dia L. Michels

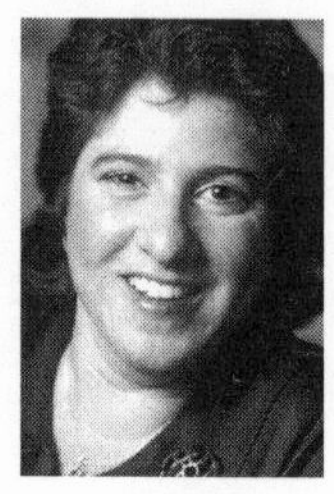

Where can families find great books in which youngsters are worn, babies are put to the breast, and children sleep with their parents? Where can mothers discover how to breastfeed after surgery and fathers learn about the environmental consequences of formula production? Where can children explore different ways families get along? In the pages of books published by Platypus Media.

As a parent, you know how important it is for children to have a loving, secure start in life. You are giving your children that start by showing them every day, in every way, that you are there for them. We share your commitment to unconditional love in early childhood as the foundation for optimal physical and mental development.

Breastfeeding, baby-wearing and family sharing are a big part of what is now labeled an attachment family. And we also know that attachment parenting values extend far beyond infancy. Support for attachment parenting concepts and behaviors is needed not only by grown-ups, but also by the children in attachment families. That's why our books include titles for infants, toddlers, preschoolers, and elementary and middle-school children - as well as our adult book on breastfeeding. As your children grow and better understand the world around them, they can appreciate these values more and more.

Each book has been created with attachment families in mind, but also for any reader who wants to share the joy of healthy childhood development and family growth. I hope you will find as much pleasure in reading and re-reading these books as we have in bringing them to you!

ORDER EXTRA COPIES
BREASTFEEDING ANNUAL INTERNATIONAL 2001

This single volume guide to the issues that surround breastfeeding policy in the fields of public health, family medicine, workplace policy and the law is an invaluable reference. The book is available through our website, platypusmedia.com or with the order form here.

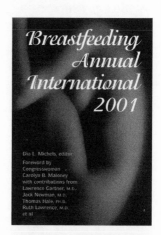

Coming In January 2003
BREASTFEEDING ANNUAL INTERNATIONAL 2003

Order your copies in advance of BREASTFEEDING ANNUAL 2003. This second edition in the series from Platypus Media features articles on breastfeeding and infectious diseases; breastfeeding after surgery; nutritional breakthroughs that affect breastfeeding choices.

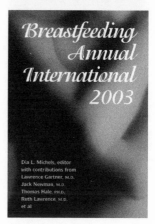

Order your Platypus Media products today.

- At our website: **PlatypusMedia.com.**
- At bookstores, catalogs, and retail websites
- Directly from us, at: **Platypus Media L.L.C.**
  627 A Street, NE,
  Washington, DC 20002 USA
  202.546.1674 or toll-free at
  877.PLATYPS (877.752.8977)
  Info@PlatypusMedia.com
  FAX 202.546.2356

North American Shipping Rates :

Ground:	$3.00 per order	+ $1.00 per item
3-Day:	$7.00 per order	+ $2.00 per item
Overnight:	$11.00 per order	+ $3.00 per item

Additional shipping information (including Canadian, International and Bulk) is available at 877-752-8977 or our website PlatypusMedia.com.

Bill to / Ship to

NAME ______________________________

ADDRESS ______________________________

____

TELEPHONE ______________________ EMAIL ______________________

If shipping to a different address, please include each name and street address on a separate piece of paper.

____ copies of *Breastfeeding Annual International 2001* BAA1 $25.95
____ copies of *Breastfeeding Annual International 2003* BAA2 $25.95

Subtotal $__________

Tax (DC residents add 6%) $__________

Shipping (see above) $__________

Grand Total $__________

Coupon or Discount code _______

Make check or money order payable to **Platypus Media**
or pay by credit card:

☐ Mastercard ☐ Visa ☐ Discover ☐ American Express

NUMBER ______________________ EXPIRATION ______________

AUTHORIZED CARDHOLDER SIGNATURE ______________________

Do you want your books autographed? If so, please tell us the name of the recipient for each title.

☐ Please send me a Platypus Media catalog